Health and Health Promoti

The impact of the United Nations "Healthy Prisons" initiative has highlighted the importance of health and health promotion in incarcerated populations. This invaluable book discusses the many health and medical issues that arise or are introduced into prisons from the perspective of both inmates and prison staff.

Health and Health Promotion in Prisons places key issues in prison health care into a historical perspective and investigates contemporary policy drivers. It then addresses the significant legal issues relating to health in prison settings and the human rights implications and questions that arise. The book presents a useful framework for health education in prison and a model for introducing structural, policy and health-related changes based on the UN Health in Prisons model, and also includes a special chapter on mental health issues.

Providing a comprehensive and thought-provoking overview of health promotion issues in correctional environments, this is an essential reference for all those involved in prison health care.

Michael W. Ross is Professor of Public Health at the University of Texas, USA.

Routledge Studies in Public Health

Health and Health Promotion in Prisons

Michael W. Ross

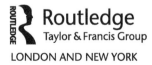

Routledge
Taylor & Francis Group

LONDON AND NEW YORK

First published 2013
by Routledge

2 Park Square, Milton Park, Abingdon, Oxon OX14 4RN
711 Third Avenue, New York, NY 10017, USA

Routledge is an imprint of the Taylor & Francis Group, an informa business

First issued in paperback 2017

British Library Cataloguing in Publication Data
A catalogue record for this book is available from the British Library

Library of Congress Cataloging-in-Publication Data
Ross, Michael W., 1952-
Health and health promotion in prisons / Michael Ross.
p. cm. -- (Routledge studies in public health)
Includes bibliographical references.
1. Prisoners--Medical care. 2. Prisoners--Health and hygiene. I. Title.
II. Series: Routledge studies in public health.
[DNLM: 1. Delivery of Health Care. 2. Prisons. 3. Health Promotion.
HV 8833]
HV8833.R67 2013
365'.667--dc23
2012017490

ISBN13: 978-0-415-52352-3 (hbk)
ISBN13: 978-1-138-10876-9 (pbk)

Typeset in Sabon
by Saxon Graphics Ltd, Derby

Contents

Foreword

I feel very honored that Professor Michael Ross should have invited me to write this foreword. He is an expert on this important subject and my understanding of the issues he explores is based largely on my experience as Her Majesty's Chief Inspector of Prisons for England and Wales between 1995 and 2001. But, having also looked at the provision of health care in prisons in the United States, Canada, many Caribbean islands, both independent and Overseas Territories, Australia, and Germany, I still remember how shaken I, as a former regular soldier and sometime chairman of an acute hospital trust, was by the appalling low standard of health care I found during my first inspection – of the largest women's prison in England – and my determination to improve it. Having read it, I just wish that this book had been available before I set out on that journey.

Professor Ross has much to say about conditions in the United Kingdom, so I do not need to describe them. My principal surprise in 1995 was to find that, uniquely, health care in prisons was not the responsibility of the National Health Service (NHS), to which every prisoner belonged before entering prison, and to which they returned. Apparently, when the NHS was established in 1947, the Prison Service claimed that, as it already had a health service, it did not need to join. That this was allowed to continue showed that neither successive governments, nor the Prison Service, appreciated the truism that Professor Ross states in the opening sentence of his book: "Prisons, jails and other correctional settings are a part of our community." Had that been recognized, health care provision within them should have been the same as that in the community. One side-effect of the situation was that there was no way of ensuring that the quality of treatment in prisons was equal to that in the community, because oversight of NHS standard did not apply.

It soon dawned on me that the mental and physical health of prisoners was a public health issue, because almost every prisoner would leave prison and therefore their state of health at that time mattered to the public to whom they were returning. If this logic had been applied, the state, which was responsible for their imprisonment, should have appreciated that it was also responsible for ensuring that, as far as humanly possible, all those whom it imprisoned returned to the community in no worse state of health that when they left. But it also dawned on me that this way by no means the sum of the state's responsibility.

The mental and physical health of every prisoner is usually checked as part of the normal procedures on reception. Because, as Professor Ross points out, so many prisoners come from what sociologists call an "underclass" of those who rarely use health facilities except in emergencies, it is inevitable that many will be found to have problems, particularly mental health problems, that have previously been unidentified or untreated. What I found in 1995 was that, largely due to lack of resources, because of the difficulty in recruiting suitable staff outside the NHS, many of these were ignored during their time in prison, with the result that prisoners were discharged into the community in a worse state of health than when they went to prison. Had health care in prisons been accepted as a public health issue, this should have been seen as being totally against the public interest, let alone the future well-being of the prisoner. How much better if time in prison was seen as an opportunity for treating, or beginning to treat, identified problems, in the public interest.

This led me to my thinking that the position of prisons in the Criminal Justice System is analogous to that of hospitals in a health service. They are the acute part, to which you should only be sent if you need the expensive treatment that only prisons or hospitals can provide. The treatment will not be completed in either prison or hospital, but will have to be continued in the community in the form of aftercare. Just as hospitals would collapse if choked with those who do not need hospital treatment, so prisons become ineffective if overcrowded with offenders who do not need to be imprisoned. If the aim of imprisonment is to protect the public by preventing reoffending, by helping those committed by the courts to live responsible and law-abiding lives in prisons and on release, then every available moment of imprisonment should be used to tackle whatever has been identified as preventing that from happening and leading to crime. Physical and, particularly, mental health problems feature largely in this, which makes it even more important that the provision of health care is of the standard required. To cut a long story short, the NHS was made responsible for prison health care in 2003, seven years after I had recommended it.

I know that the same conditions do not apply in the United States, but, as Professor Ross describes so clearly, the same thought process regarding the promotion and provision of a proper standard of health care, and understanding and satisfying the issues he examines, apply anywhere and everywhere in the world. Prisons should not be exempt from national initiatives, such as "Healthy People 2010." The health of prisoners, while in prison and on discharge, is a matter of public interest, and therefore public health, wherever anyone is held in prison. To satisfy doubters, in addition to exploring the moral and human rights issues connected with the promotion of decent health care, Ross goes on to describe and examine the issues at the heart of its provision itself. Prison health care may not be regarded as a mainstream activity within a health service, nor nurses and health care assistants automatically as full members of custodial staff teams. But those responsible must understand all the issues that the promotion of health care involves, including accepting that it must be carried out by fully trained professionals.

There will always be a selection of the public who feel that criminals should be locked in their cells and the key thrown away; it is unfortunate that such views enjoy undue prominence in our sensation- and circulation-obsessed media. If the media bosses read Professor Ross' book they might realize that such attitudes are the antithesis of the protection of the public because of what prisons can do to protect the public if properly resourced. I hope therefore that it will be widely read, particularly by those responsible for health promotion and therefore public health in prisons.

David Ramsbotham
London
March 2012

Acknowledgments

This is not the book I started writing. I was intending to write a summary of public health issues in jails and prisons, but shortly afterwards an excellent edited volume came out which it made no sense to duplicate. It was at that point that I decided to start writing on issues that I thought defined public health, and particularly health promotion, in prisons, and to let the book "write itself." The result is this volume on history, health promotion, law and human rights, infectious diseases and occupational health and safety in correctional settings. I have focused on the two systems which I have some understanding of – the US and the English and Welsh systems – which have their similarities and differences, and advantages and disadvantages.

I also intended to write this book for other academics, but the more I wrote, the more I recalled my thesis advisor at the University of Cambridge, Professor Alison Liebling, commenting that if one wanted to write for the audience that was among the most influential, one should write for prison officers. I have therefore written a book that I hope will be readable by both prison custodial and health staff and the educated lay public (including correctional consumers), and by policy-makers in the penal area, as well as by academics and students. It will probably please none of these, because public health and health promotion in prisons is a totally interactive field: what affects staff affects inmates, and vice versa. It can only be approached by considering it an integrated system influenced by history, philosophy, education, law, administration and policy, and of course medicine and public health.

My greatest debt of gratitude is to my teachers at the Institute of Criminology at the University of Cambridge: Professor Alison Liebling, whose ground-breaking work on prisons and moral performance has influenced my thinking enormously; Sir Tony Bottoms, Shadd Maruna, Tim Coupe and my teachers in the Masters degree in criminology; and particularly to my teacher and tutor Nicky Padfield at the Faculty of Law, University of Cambridge, whose wisdom and guidance have greatly influenced my thinking and writing. While I still don't think and write like a lawyer, I hope I have come some way toward understanding the legal issues involved in prison health, and certainly I am fascinated by them. While any mistakes are my own, many have been avoided by Nicky's very constructive criticisms (usually prefaced by the phrase "Well, I'm just a simple lawyer, *but...*"). My prison governor and officer colleagues at Cambridge have also encouraged me to see issues practically and from both sides of the staff–inmate divide, and to realize that this divide is in many ways a very arbitrary one. My graduate students at the University of Texas could also be counted on to ask tough questions on areas I hadn't thought about.

My friends and colleagues Drs. Ruth Armstrong (University of Cambridge) and Pam Diamond and Amy Jo Harzke (University of Texas) gave encouragement, guidance, editing advice and references to literature I might otherwise have missed, and imposed logic where it was lacking. To the extent that this is readable, they are to be thanked. Dr. Amy Jo Harzke also co-wrote Chapter 8 with me. The WHO Prisons Project in Europe was a source of inspiration and a model of how health and prisons could be integrated.

This book would not have got off the ground without a generous sabbatical leave from the School of Public Health, University of Texas, to work back at the Institute of Criminology, University of Cambridge, and to the welcoming environment of Fitzwilliam College at Cambridge. The Institute of Criminology librarians, Mary Gower and Stuart Stone, were also a source of enormous help during my time there. Finally, I am enormously grateful to David, Lord Ramsbotham, whose approach as Chief Inspector of Prisons in England and Wales inspired me to attempt to write about prison health from a broad perspective rather than from the narrowly medical, and who has generously contributed the foreword to this book.

1 The need for correctional public health and health promotion

Prisons, jails and other correctional settings are a part of the community. They also serve to focus risk for many diseases, either by concentrating people with elevated risks, or by providing the conditions for exacerbation or transmission of some diseases. And, as part of the community, they return the vast majority of inmates back into the community. Thus, correctional public health and health promotion is arguably of as much, if not more, significance than "free world" community health. In correctional settings, people with actual or potentially elevated risks are concentrated and probably easier to screen, treat and educate than those in the community. This introduction is not intended to be an exhaustive review of health in prisons: for that, there are excellent texts available (for example, Greifinger, 2010). Its purpose is to introduce the significance of health and disease in prisons and the opportunities it provides for interventions. I have chosen to emphasize data for one US state, Texas, as an example, in addition to wider US data, simply to make the point that even in a single statewide community, there are major issues with prison and jail health and major opportunities to address them. If, as former Speaker of the US House of Representatives Tip O'Neill once said, "All politics is local," then ultimately all health is local – and personal – too.

Public health risks and social disadvantage

Disease in society follows a process of social sedimentation. Poor health and disease, whether communicable or chronic, is more prevalent in those with lower income, education and occupation, and this relationship holds in the United States within racial/ethnic groups, as well as between them. Further, this relationship is compounded by Hart's (1971) Inverse Care Law, which notes that those with the greatest burden of disease have the least access to health services (including preventive health programs), and vice versa. However, the sedimentation of disease, where the highest rates are found in the lowest levels of society, is not solely a function of availability and utilization of services. If issues of disease, particularly communicable diseases, are to be dealt with in those "core transmission groups" in the community where rates are highest and where utilization of services is lowest, then correctional institutions (jails, prisons, juvenile and other detention facilities) and their populations are central to disease reduction efforts. Core groups are those responsible for most of the transmission of STDs: it has been estimated that more than 80 percent of STDs are transmitted by less than 20 percent of the population (Yorke *et al.*, 1978). Further, Okie (2007) estimates that each year, 25 percent of people with HIV in the United States will spend time in a correctional facility, as will 33 percent of people with Hepatitis C.

Health risks and social disadvantage among correctional populations

The population who circulate through correctional institutions (prisons, jails, juvenile detention centers and other specialist correctional units such as substance abuse felony punishment units) form a significant part of an "underclass" (a sociological term for those who are frequently marginalized, unemployed, on welfare or other assistance, in persistent poverty, have significant barriers to health care and may have a family history of more than one generation in this situation), who are difficult to access and who rarely use available health facilities except in emergencies. Reduction or elimination of most communicable diseases is not possible without a focus on the lowest levels of society in terms of income, education and occupation, and correctional institutions are a key to accessing, treating and preventing disease transmission in this population. In this context, as Virchow (1941) noted, "The physicians are the natural attorneys of the poor, and social problems fall to a large extent within their jurisdiction." Preventive innovations may diffuse from inmates to their families and associates, both in terms of preventive behaviors and of lowered disease transmission rates, making diffusion of information to other at-risk members of the community a positive additional impact, as well as making those treated *de facto* peer educators in their communities.

Medical conditions among incarcerated populations

In 2009, Binswanger *et al.* looked at nationally representative data from surveys of inmates in the United States. Even with adjustment for important sociodemographic differences including sex, age, race, education, employment, US birth, marital status and alcohol consumption, jail and prison inmates had a higher burden of most chronic conditions. Binswanger *et al.* report that compared with the general population, prison and jail inmates had higher rates (odds ratios [ORs] given for jail first and prison second) for hypertension (OR = 1.19, 1.17); asthma (OR = 1.41, 1.34); arthritis (OR = 1.65, 1.66); cervical cancer (OR = 4.16, 4.82); and Hepatitis (OR = 2.57, 4.23). There was no increased risk for diabetes, angina or myocardial infarction, and lower odds of obesity. These data were based on self-report and so may be underestimates of conditions which were not clinically obvious or had not been diagnosed. These data emphasize the chronic, as well as infectious, conditions that are over-represented in correctional populations.

Prevention and public health for communicable diseases in correctional institutions involves reducing staff risk as well as inmate risk

Correctional institutions need to be targeted in terms of both inmates and staff, since for communicable diseases such as meningococcal infections, influenza, pneumococcal infections, tuberculosis (TB), and Hepatitis A, B/D and C, among others, spread between inmates and staff, and from staff to their families and the outside community, is not limited. In this sense, the concept of inmates as being part of a closed community for disease transmission is inappropriate. A recent study in Texas found that over one-quarter of men and nearly half of women entering the Texas Department of Criminal Justice system were infected with Hepatitis C (Baillargeon *et al.*, 2003). Attention needs to be equally given to the health of correctional staff and service providers. While correctional institutions are designed, among other purposes, to provide protection to society from those incarcerated, they do this only physically. From the point of infectious diseases, they provide almost no protection, with staff and the community almost as much at risk as if the offenders were in the wider community. Indeed, the level of risk may be greater because of the concentration of "at risk" groups in incarcerated settings. Prevention, including immunization where available, thus becomes a matter of occupational as well as public safety.

Endpoints for interventions with the incarcerated might include risk reduction among "high risk" groups, reducing risk for correctional staff and their families (including vaccination where appropriate) and reducing risk between inmates and their social networks post-release. All of these endpoints can be addressed in prison- or jail-based health programs.

An important component of public health surveillance and screening

For communicable diseases, correctional facilities are a key – but often neglected – component of surveillance, screening, treatment and prevention. The burden of disease is extremely high in the correctional population: 35 percent of TB, over 50 percent of Hepatitis C, and in 1996, 17 percent of HIV cases were detected in people passing through correctional facilities. Over one-quarter of new syphilis cases and very significant numbers of cases of gonorrhea and chlamydia are identified in correctional facilities. There are up to 45,000 cases of HIV infection currently in US correctional facilities.

Core transmitters for many of the most significant communicable diseases pass through prisons and jails, and any attempt to reduce disease burden thus needs to focus on correctional populations. Risser *et al.* (2001) found that 10 percent of males and 18 percent of females in a juvenile detention center in Houston were infected with chlamydia, and 88 percent of these were treated while incarcerated. Prisons and jails get many of the disease prevention failures from the wider community, but can then function as a safety net to treat or prevent transmission if there are adequate public health programs developed for correctional populations. It is likely that adequate prevention efforts in the correctional setting would have a disproportionately large impact on the free world community's health and communicable disease prevalence. Binswanger *et al.* (2005) found that jail could also be an appropriate venue in which to provide cancer screening for a high-risk population, especially for African American and other minority populations, and for breast and colon cancer screening.

High health and death risks on immediate release from prison

In recent evidence, Binswanger *et al.* (2007) conducted a comprehensive study on deaths of released inmates in Washington State and found that risk of death in the 1.9 years after release was 3.5 times higher than in other state residents, after adjusting for age, race/ethnicity and sex. In the first two weeks after release, the death of former inmates was over 12 times that of other state residents! The most elevated risk (129 times that of state residents) was of death from drug overdose. Binswanger *et al.* report that in addition to high vulnerability to drug overdose, in the two weeks following release, risk of death from violence, unintended injury, and a lapse in treatment of chronic health conditions is also high (and significantly higher for females than males). In Houston, Harzke *et al.* (2006) studied prisoners receiving HIV treatment in state prisons, and despite post-release incentives, half of the inmates were lost to follow-up and did not access or maintain their antiretroviral medications following release. This has serious implications not only for the former inmates, but for the development (and transmission from those former inmates) of drug-resistant forms of HIV. Former inmates with stable housing and who did not use alcohol post-release were most likely to access primary care. Risser and Smith (2005) similarly note for TB in incarcerated youth in Texas that less than 10 percent kept follow-up appointments or continued their treatment. Transitional medical care post-release for many infectious or chronic conditions may be critical, not only for the former inmate, but also for transmission to the public of infectious conditions (possibly drug-resistant) such as HIV, TB, and Hepatitis B and C. Good public and community health involves managing the transition from prison to community as seamlessly as possible to ensure that any gains from prison interventions are not lost by lack of maintenance or treatment on return to the community or in fact by higher risk of death or relapse.

Health risk interventions with correctional populations

One of the major goals of the "Healthy People 2010" ten-year health objectives of the US Federal Government (US Department of Health and Human Services, 2000) was the reduction of racial and ethnic disparities in health, particularly including those in HIV/AIDS, STDs and immunizations. Correctional institutions provide an important venue for education, screening and prevention activities in the United States and should be a focus of these aspects of the ten-year plan. Conklin *et al.* (1998) note that in a large northeastern correctional facility, for example, 82 percent of inmates reported no history of a regular medical provider at time of incarceration, and 93 percent had no form of medical insurance. Clearly, inmates are not likely to be served by traditional medical and public health services. Correctional facilities, therefore, can play a significant role in reducing both disease burden and risk behaviors. Further, as emergency rooms in large metropolitan areas are overburdened with walk-in non-emergency care cases from the under-served and "underclass" populations, an emphasis on screening and prevention in correctional facilities could have a cost-effective impact on inappropriate use of expensive emergency room services. However, as Harzke *et al.* (2006) noted for released inmates with HIV, only half in their Texas sample were in primary care three weeks after release, and thus half were not continuing medication.

Preventing disease transmission within correctional environments

In addition to holding inmates with communicable diseases, some correctional environments also provide opportunities for activities that transmit disease. Wolfe *et al.* (2001) describe a major outbreak of syphilis in three prisons in the south of the United States, and they note that in most institutions, inmates are not isolated but are inescapably, from the perspective of infectious diseases, part of the American community. This is inevitable, they argue, given the movement of detainees through jail, prison and the community, and most inmates return to the community, bringing with them infectious diseases harbored or acquired through correctional facilities. HIV has also been recorded as spreading in correctional facilities (Mutter *et al.*, 1994). Despite intentions of staff, and state laws notwithstanding, risk behavior exists at high levels in correctional facilities, whether sexual activity, use of smuggled drugs or "home brew" alcohol, injecting or tattooing, or poor diet or opportunities for exercise.

Correctional populations comprise a significant proportion of the US population, particularly young African American males (Osemene *et al.*, 2001), and an even more significant proportion of the population that carries the greatest burden of preventable and treatable communicable diseases. In 2000, the total estimated US correctional population (prison, jail, probation, parole) was 6,467,200, plus an additional 105,790 juveniles in detention. In Texas, as an example of one of the largest states, the figure at the same time was slightly over 150,000, or 1 in 20 adults in the state. This constitutes nearly 4 percent of the adult population of the country, and 5 percent in Texas. The Texas Department of Criminal Justice is the second largest correctional service in the United States, and one of the largest in the world. As of August 31, 2006, total receives were over 74,000 (62,804 males and 11,366 females), with nearly 26,000 African American and 26,000 White inmates, and over 22,000 Hispanic inmates. These were divided between prison (43,138) and state jail (25,690), with the remainder in youth programs. The majority (34,871) were in minimum custody, and mean sentence length was 8.5 years (of which average time served was 4.5 years) for the prison inmates (0.8 years is the mean sentence length for state jail inmates) (Texas Department of Criminal Justice, 2006). Two in three prison inmates will return to prison within three years of first release (*Sourcebook of Criminal Justice Statistics*, 2001).

Effective evaluation of correctional health promotion programs

Some correctional systems have innovative programs set in correctional environments that deserve evaluation and wider dissemination. For example, the Texas HIV prevention curriculum uses peer educators to teach and disseminate information about HIV prevention and reaches a large population including not just inmates, but their families and other contacts in the "free world." Ross *et al.* (2006) evaluated this program and found it to be highly effective across inmates of varying educational and socioeconomic backgrounds, and to result in increased HIV testing in inmates who had been exposed to it. Mullen *et al.* (2003) have described many of the constraints in carrying out public health interventions, such as their alcohol-exposed pregnancy prevention program in a women's county jail in Texas, which make it clear that conducting public health interventions in a correctional setting requires modifications to adapt them to jail operational needs and policies, staff limitations and inmate perceptions, as well as follow-up difficulties post-release. Understanding and adapting to setting and target group constraints in correctional contexts requires careful design, preparation and evaluation, and public health specialists familiar with these constraints (Mullen *et al.*, 2003). It also requires appropriate buy-in, and a joint collaboration, including joint planning, between correctional staff, health care staff and public health specialists. Without a shared commitment and interest from all sectors (including administration, inmates and staff), health-related programs in correctional settings are predestined to failure.

High through-flow and opportunity for public health interventions in correctional facilities

Contrary to popular perception, most stays in correctional facilities are relatively short. For example, in Houston (Harris County Jail), Texas, the mean stay is 34 days, and over 7,000 inmates are released each month. This pattern is typical of urban areas in the United States. For the Texas Department of Criminal Justice, the average prison inmate serves 4.5 years of an average 8.5-year sentence and has an eighth-grade education; the prison population turnover is about one-third per year. In the United States there are approximately 12.5 million adult correctional facility entries and 12 million exits per year, approaching 10 percent of the adult population. About 45 percent of those released return to prison within five months, and thus there is a cycling between correctional institutions and the community comprising people who are not only at the highest risk for communicable diseases, but also are not usually seeking or accessing care in any place. Public health programs in correctional facilities could have a very significant impact on the communicable disease burden in the United States by accessing the population where the attributable risk is extremely high. Further, this population is commonly not accessible through other health care programs, and are accessible, sober and without competing interests while in correctional facilities. Correctional institutions, for many of their population, are a "revolving door" to the community, with jail inmates returning faster and in larger numbers and thus having more of an impact on community health (Mullen *et al.*, 2003). Correctional health in the field of communicable diseases is thus clearly not only a matter of considerable significance for community health, but also of public safety: for communicable diseases, incarceration is not, and cannot be considered, quarantine from the wider population.

Organizational and health interactions

There is a close relationship between health in prisons and prison organization and facilities. In a review of the Greek prison system, Cheliotis (2012) reports that prison establishments are vastly overcrowded and conditions of detainment are deplorable, with minimal health care provision and high prevalence of serious transmissible diseases, mental disorders, deliberate self-harm and suicide and death. He notes that the harms of imprisonment are typically centered upon two central issues: physical conditions and prisoner health. In Greece, the rise of the prison population is largely accounted for by an increase in drug-related offences (over 30 percent of convicted prisoners) and non-Greek offenders (over 40 percent of convicted prisoners, the majority of whom are Albanian). One consequence of this overcrowding is that over one-third of prisoners reported deliberate self-harm in prison, including hitting one's own head, wrist-cutting and self-burning, all correlated with overcrowded conditions. Suicides were highest in overcrowded facilities and dropped dramatically in semi-open and agricultural prisons. Creation of poor health through prison conditions can and does occur.

Gross overcrowding in Greek prisons is exacerbated by most of the health-related posts being unfilled, by the criterion of the number of health care posts provided by the relevant Act (a number arguably itself too meager for prisoner needs and based on lower numbers of inmates). Only 39 percent of needed health care staff are in place, including only 22 percent of medical staff and the same proportion of dentists; only half of the nursing positions are filled. This is in a country with an *oversupply* of medical and dental specialists and pharmacists! Staffing is so low that most health care centers in prisons are run by prison officers and prisoners themselves, Cheliotis notes. There was one prisoner death every ten days (including suicide, drug overdose and other causes). It is clear from the Greek example that health conditions in prisons are intimately associated with the prison organization, level of staffing, overcrowding and physical environment, and that it is often difficult to disentangle these interactions since they are all due to official neglect and disinterest.

The relationship of health services to prison climate was investigated by Ross *et al.* (2011) in 49 English and Welsh correctional institutions. They were able to be more specific about the mechanisms and conditions that were associated with inmates' health care satisfaction in the Measuring the Quality of Prison Life (MQPL) instrument. Interestingly, the prison climate dimensions of *relationships with staff, safety, feedback and care, fairness* and *care for the vulnerable* predicted one-third of the variance in health care satisfaction of inmates. Clearly, health care provision and access are an integral part of prison climate and specifically of non-health-related aspects of climate. Ross *et al.*'s data suggested that positive prison climates – which are characterized by positive prisoner–staff interaction, fairness and care for the vulnerable – are also likely to have the best health care provision and access. This, they speculate, is likely because prison staff are crucial gatekeepers between the cells and the clinic. A negative prison climate may also contaminate the ethical and care-giving standards of prison health care staff and the organizational aspects of prisoner health care; for example, the provision of health-related case conferences between prison staff and health care staff. Further, because prison health care depends on prison staff identifying and facilitating health interventions where there is illness or distress, the moral climate of the prison plays a major part in ensuring access to care before conditions reach extremes of distress or severity. As Ross *et al.* note, in institutions with poor prison climates, health care tends to be negligent or substandard. Thus, general prison moral and organizational climate impacts health care as an integral part of the institution and its ethos.

Conclusions

There are good reasons from both public and community health standpoints, as well as from the point of occupational health and safety, to focus on correctional health as one area where there is high "bang for the buck" in reducing the burden of disease in the community. Our reluctance to provide for such services stems partly from a psychological distaste for providing for people we cannot readily identify with, partly from philosophical distaste for providing services for those who we see as needing punishment, and partly from the fact that correctional populations may contain a significant proportion of people who it is difficult and often challenging to work with. None of these reasons justifies ignoring the problem. That is not to say that working with correctional populations is necessarily easy or glamorous, but it is part of the web of community health care and of truly national programs which have health for all as their desired outcome. It cannot be ignored. Nor can we assume that a narrow focus on health without looking at legal, political and policy, philosophical, economic and organizational (including environmental and occupational health) factors will be adequate. Indeed, some of the greatest barriers to adequate and effective correctional health are much broader than the health agenda and must be addressed before much progress will be made.

2 Health in prisons

A historical perspective

> Many who went in healthy, are in a few months changed to emaciated, dejected objects. Some are seen pining under diseases, "sick, and in prison"; expiring on the floors, in loathsome cells, of pestilential fevers, and the confluent smallpox.
>
> Howard, 1784, p. 1

Historically, health in jails and prisons has always been a major issue. The combination of keeping large numbers of people in small, confined spaces with poor ventilation and little light, often chained together or to a wall, and with poor nutrition, is a recipe for ill health or death and the development of epidemics. Further, there was usually no incentive to keep prisoners alive and healthy unless they were state prisoners of high rank, or were imprisoned awaiting a ransom. In such latter cases, or where the prisoner's family and friends were able to pay the jailor to ensure their survival in good health, there were economic incentives to improve conditions.

The danger of dying in prison from the effects of the prison environment on health was always real. An edict of the Roman Emperor Constantine the Great (AD 272–337) notes the risk that inmates "perish from the torments of prison" (Peters, 1995, p. 20), from the single or combined effects of overcrowding, filth, chains and starvation. Indeed, the torments of prison were a source of compulsion for prisoners' families and friends to pay the jailor to ameliorate their conditions, and for imprisoned debtors or those awaiting ransom to make payment as quickly as possible. Jailors' fees might include a "suavitas" (literally, "charm") to buy more pleasant treatment, and "iron fees" to ensure lighter or minimal chains (Peters, 1995, p. 35). Jailors were usually paid minimally or irregularly, if at all, and were expected to recoup their expenses from prisoners.

Prisons as short-term holding facilities

While punitive imprisonment was an option in most ancient and medieval systems, it was usually in the form of coercive imprisonment of limited duration, and in the case of debtors was designed to encourage payment. Usually, capital punishment or exile was the preferred sentence, since punitive imprisonment was at the cost of the state and thus not encouraged. In the Roman Empire, private imprisonment for household members and slaves was a prerogative of the household head (Peters, 1995).

Monastic and religious prisons introduced more widespread punitive imprisonment, but civil law in Europe tended to favor imprisonment only until trial occurred, and then various immediate forms of punishment such as death or mutilation, public shaming or loss of property, with punitive imprisonment rare because of cost. In Italy in the twelfth century, fines began to be combined with imprisonment. Peters (1995), along with Spierenburg (1995), suggests that the development of the modern prison in the eighteenth and nineteenth centuries was part of a movement toward "lesser punishments" than public torture and death, perhaps with a view to correction as well as punishment. The first significant use of workhouses occurred in the early 1600s in western Europe. These were organized around penal servitude, as was transportation to colonies for forced labor as these sites became available to Britain and France in the Americas, and after 1776 (when the independence of the American colonies made it necessary to find other destinations for transportation) to Australia. Spierenburg notes that in Britain, even in the third quarter of the eighteenth century, only about one-tenth of convicts were sentenced to imprisonment.

Prisons as foci for morbidity and mortality

Conditions in jails and prisons changed little up to the late eighteenth century. McConville (1995, p. 307) quotes William Smith, a doctor who visited the London jails in the mid-1770s and who described prisoners as

> vagrants and disorderly women of the very lowest and most wretched class of human beings, almost naked with only a few filthy rags almost alive and in motion with vermin, their bodies rotting with the bad distemper, and covered in itch, scorbutic and venereal ulcers.

Here, Smith identifies several diseases common to prisoners. While "distemper" was a general term for illness at the time, scorbutic ulcers were a consequence of scurvy (vitamin C deficiency arising from inadequate diet, delaying wound healing and fatal in extreme cases). Venereal ulcers probably refer to syphilitic ulcers, primary chancres at the site of infection, and more generally to yaws, a very similar treponemal infection which is epidemic. It may also refer to gummata, erosions of the connective tissue down to the bone, which are a symptom of tertiary syphilis. From Smith's description, prison was an extremely unhealthy place to be.

John Howard's definitive *The State of the Prisons* (1784) is a detailed description of prisons in the United Kingdom and across Europe. Howard

(1784, p. xix–xx) observes that prison may frequently be a death sentence, reporting from records that in the King's Bench (London) prison alone in the six years prior to 1579, 100 prisoners died of disease. In the 1770s, he also records the deaths from "gaol-fever and the smallpox, which I saw prevailing to the destruction of multitudes, not only of felons in their dungeons, but of debtors also." Gaol (jail)-fever is typhus, a lice-borne disease caused by the *Rikettsia* bacterium and characterized by high fevers and headaches: untreated, it may have a mortality of only 20 percent in healthy individuals, but up to 60 percent in the elderly or the debilitated. The headaches progress to delirium and death. It is spread rapidly by human body lice and was responsible for enormous death tolls in prisons and concentration camps, exacerbated by starvation and crowding. In England, "imprisonment until the next term of court" was considered a death sentence. Howard also noted similar epidemics in European prisons (1784, p. 124). Of his visit in Pampalona, Spain, he records that "epidemical distempers" had recently prevailed, killing 18 of 20 prisoners in a short time.

Typhus was no respecter of class or role: there are a number of descriptions of epidemics killing court and prison staff as well as prisoners. At the Oxford Assize (later referred to as the "Black Assize") of 1577, 300 died, including the lord chief baron, and at the Taunton Assize of 1730, the lord chief baron, the high sheriff, the sergeant and hundreds of others also died. Howard (1784, p. 153) records the death of a gaol physician of gaol-fever, and of the keeper and his wife at Launceston dying of gaol-fever in one night (p. 391), along with many prisoners. Howard himself died of typhus while visiting prisons in the Ukraine in 1790.

Models of disease and their implications for prison health

Howard's work in the early 1770s led to the introduction and passing of an "Act for Preserving the Health of Prisoners and Preventing Gaol-Distemper," introduced into the House of Commons by Alexander Popham, MP for Taunton, and passed into law in 1774. This bill, in keeping with the prevailing view of the causation of disease, laid the blame for disease in prison on "want of cleanliness and fresh air" (Howard, 1784, p. xx). Until the late 1800s, disease was perceived as being caused by dirt and bad air. Early physicians made the epidemiological connection between fevers and low-lying areas by rivers and marshes: indeed, the bad air (in Italian, "mal aria") that arose from such sites was blamed for fevers that we now know to be mosquito-borne, such as malaria, yellow fever and dengue. The higher burden of disease among the poor, who lived in the lower areas with poor drainage and close to the discharge of sewage into rivers and other watercourses, which were also mosquito breeding grounds, was blamed on the poor air. These observations on the *distribution* of disease by class and geography were correct, but the explanation, although logical from the data, we now know to be incorrect. Infectious causes began to be suspected after John Snow's studies of the London cholera epidemic showed that the disease was associated not with the air, but with use of particular water sources. His famous removal of the pump handle of the Broad Street pump in 1854, leading to the cessation of the cholera epidemic in the part of the city served by that pump (which drew water from downstream of the sewage outfall), demonstrated the accuracy of his theory of water-borne diseases.

Environmental conditions, specifically bad air and dirt, were regarded as causing disease until the work of Pasteur and Koch in the late 1860s and 1870s demonstrated that bacteria and other organisms were the cause of infectious diseases (a theory that took several decades to become fully accepted). In the late 1800s, understanding of disease transmission was further expanded by the work of Ronald Ross, which established that insects were also vectors of disease (notably, the mosquito for transmission of malaria) and shortly thereafter the work of Carlos Finlay and Walter Reed in Cuba, which also identified the mosquito as the vector for yellow fever. Thus, our reading of the history of health in prisons up to the late 1800s needs to be on the basis of the *prevailing* and commonly accepted theories of infection. Howard himself indicated that he avoided becoming infected by changing his clothes after visiting prisons (cleanliness, which would also reduce the carriage of lice) and constantly smelling vinegar while in the prison (to counteract the bad air – but vinegar is also an effective antiseptic). Frequent lime-washing of rooms (Howard recommended twice-yearly: "The rooms were very clean; they are lime-whited twice a year, and they are washed every day" [p. 178]) also served to kill parasites, and frequent changing of straw and bedding served to remove materials which could also harbor parasites such as lice and ticks and materials that could attract rodents, themselves carrying fleas that might transmit disease. The use of vinegar, and lime as wash, were an effective antiseptic and topical insecticide, although their mechanism of action was not to be understood for another century.

However, interestingly, Howard also identified infectious causes of disease, without making the leap to specific agents of disease. He reports on a number of cases where prisoners were transferred from one jail to another, or from prisons to ships, transferring disease with them, and thus were the source of epidemics (1784, pp. 7–8). He cites the work of the famous navy surgeon James Lind, who refers to the "seeds of infection." Indeed, Howard was one of the first to use this threat to the general public health of prisoners returning to their communities and bringing with them disease, to argue for prison health (an argument we tend to think of as modern). While Howard was, using Kuhn's (1970) model of the structure of scientific revolutions, working within the dirt and "miasma" (bad air) paradigm, he was also making observations that revealed some of the potential anomalies in the prevailing theory. Such anomalies would eventually lead to the infectious agent paradigm, where these "seeds" of infection were finally identified as microorganisms (protozoa, bacteria, viruses and, more recently, sub-viral particles). Nevertheless, the transmission of some air-borne diseases (for example, tuberculosis) is still consistent with parts of the "miasma" paradigm.

The work of Ignaz Semmelweis in 1847 in Austria (based on the "cleanliness" paradigm) and subsequently Lister in 1867 in England (based on the "germ" paradigm), established that physician cleanliness, through washing with antiseptics such as carbolic acid solutions, could cut post-operative patient deaths by an order of magnitude. Semmelweis demonstrated that physicians washing their hands between obstetric deliveries could cut cases of puerperal fever and subsequent maternal death from over 10 percent of deliveries to about 1–2 percent. However, he was considered insane for his arguments and died shortly after being committed to an asylum, his death apparently as a result of being beaten by the guards. In contrast, Joseph Lister, whose work in the UK 20 years later had the benefit of an acceptable scientific explanation, following as it did closely on Pasteur's demonstration of the existence of disease- and decay-causing bacteria, was created a baron by Queen Victoria.

Death rates

Howard (1784) notes that the number of prisoners dying in prison in England far exceeded the number executed in any year! The effects of confinement and infectious diseases are illustrated by the death rate of the second fleet of convicts from England to Australia in 1790, where 26 percent of the convicts died during a voyage of 160 days (and 47 percent of those who embarked were disembarked very sick). However, in the first fleet, with Captain Arthur Philip's care for the state of his ships, obtaining fresh food at each port, and provision of exercise space and adequate medical care, the death rate was about 3 percent (Hirst, 1995). The comparison between the death rates in the first and second fleets, less than three years apart, illustrates the order of magnitude of difference between good and poor care, even given the relatively inadequate medical care of the time. Howard also notes how epidemics appeared to be associated with overcrowding in prisons (p. 259).

Nevertheless, environmental conditions on their own certainly also caused death: Darlington (1955) reports that crowding of prisoners in the Marshalsea prison in London was so severe that in hot weather in the 1720s, 8–10 prisoners died every 24 hours. Extremes of temperature in prisons were themselves widely recognized as causing disability or death. In Paris, at the Cour Royale prison, Howard reports that several hundred prisoners died in the severe cold in 1775 (p. 134). In the dungeons of the St. Joseph prison at Lyons, in contrast, he noted 29 criminals "the heat so excessive, that few of them had any other garment on than their shirts" (p. 137). Crowding itself could lead to death, as he also noted in Castlebar in Ireland: "Many poor wretches have been almost suffocated in this small prison.

Forty-two prisoners have been confined in a room twenty-one feet by seventeen" (p. 156).

Howard provides precise death numbers, total prisoner numbers and time periods for death rates for prisoners of war of a number of nations in Britain from the late 1770s to the early 1780s, allowing for calculation of annual death rates. From his figures, the death rate among American prisoners was about 1.5 percent, for French prisoners 0.3 percent, for Spanish prisoners 1.8 percent and for Dutch prisoners 0.6 percent per annum. These may be similar to general population rates for young, relatively healthy men at the time, although nearly half a century later it was demonstrated that jail mortality was nearly double that of the country population of the same age (Wiener, 1995). Prisoners of war, however, could generally expect better treatment than felons or debtors.

Given often inadequate staffing levels, deaths by trauma were often reported, and there was often free access to alcohol in prisons (many jailors in British prisons also ran drinking establishments on premises and supplied alcohol to prisoners for a fee). Standley (1995) notes how the jailor at Stafford was licensed to sell beer and wine in the prison until 1784 as a means of making a living. Howard reported (in Dublin's Newgate prison) that "There are many instances of persons dying by intoxication and fighting: one lay dead when I was in the infirmary, and another was killed a few days after" (p. 154).

Nutritional inadequacies also clearly contributed to illness and death in prisons: first, by reducing the body's resistance to infection; second, by the production of nutritional deficiency diseases such as scurvy; and probably, in some instances, by actual starvation. Howard frequently refers to the importance of diet in prisoner health, and himself weighed the bread and meat rations in the prisons he visited (and often noted significant discrepancies between the weight supposed to be given and that actually given). He observes that it is impossible that "a man who lives upon bread and water can work hard and be kept in health" (p. 107). At Lille, Howard (p. 125) noted that "the scurvy has lately made great havoc here" and describes the diet as consisting of bread and small beer (low or no alcohol). The lack of vitamin C in such a diet would result in scurvy. Beer was often preferred to water as the alcohol level made it safer to drink than water (which we now understand as being due to the bacteriocidal properties of the alcohol). Poor nutrition was, however, implicated in poor wound healing in prisoners, and many prison medical officers in England tried to keep prisoners in hospital for a fortnight or three weeks before an operation if possible, to ensure post-operative wound healing. It was generally recognized that the quantity of daily nourishment was inadequate for men at hard labor (Hardy, 1995).

Occupational health and safety risks also contributed to the morbidity of prisoners. As an example, Howard (1784, p. 106) notes the unhealthy effect of the prisoners' work grinding lenses (up to 400 per week) and the "disagreeable sensations" from the dust of the lenses. However, such occupational health and safety risks were widespread throughout the population at that time and probably no worse in prisons than elsewhere. Environmental stress may also have played a part in prison health. Porter (1995, pp. 12–13) highlights Howard's belief that the sudden negative change of diet and lodging so affected the spirits of new prisoners that psychological factors, including morale, led to "sickness and despair."

Cleanliness (or filth) was noted regularly by Howard, and he correctly associated cleanliness with greater health in prisoners. However, this may have been due not only to its resulting decrease in parasites, but also because it was a marker of the level of care of prison authorities for their charges. Porter (1995) points out that for Howard, the prison sick-list was a warning signal, the symptoms of a sick institution (p. 11). Howard gives an example of a contagious disease in the Hôtel-Dieu prison in Paris:

> The cause of it was generally thought to be want of cleanliness in prisons; where several of those confined had worn their linen for many months, and infected the most healthy new-comers that were put in the room with them
>
> (p. 128)

Howard notes with approval that in 1753 a fund was set up in Paris to provide prisoners with clean linen weekly, from a stock of 5,000 shirts, and that this charity was supported by the king (Louis XV) and queen, among others. Such charities also supplied soup twice a week and meat once a fortnight, he records.

Medical care in prisons

Medical care in prisons was rudimentary, as indeed it was elsewhere in society. There was the additional barrier of the concept of "lesser entitlement" of prisoners, in addition to the cost of providing medical care to them. Standley (1995), in a detailed description of the medical treatment of prisoners in Stafford Gaol in the eighteenth century, notes that a surgeon and an apothecary were retained to treat prisoners. Such treatment included bleeding and purging transports (prisoners to be transported) before they were conveyed to Liverpool. Itemized treatment costs give an indication of the medical conditions experienced: treatment for leg abscesses and gangrene, ointment and physic for the itch, purging draughts, medicine for venereal disease, treatment for fever, dressing wounds, ointment for vermin, various bleedings and treatment for stomach disorders and piles. Quicksilver (mercury, a highly toxic treatment for syphilis) was prescribed for one man. Orders for enhanced diets may also have been given for some sick prisoners. Vinegar and soap were also provided to wash prisoners prior to trial. As Porter (1995) notes, medicine was not ready for responsibility for health until the late nineteenth century. Hardy (1995) dates the development of the

Prison Medical Service in the UK to the 1850 Act for the Better Governance of Convict Prisons. Before then, with some exceptions, treatment consisted mainly of bleeding and purging, which in many cases may have hastened death. Thus, the tension between punishment and care was minimal compared with present society, although the rule of "less eligibility" which stemmed from the fact that prisoners were there as a deterrent to further crime was applied (Sim, 1990, 1995; Wiener, 1995). As Sim notes, prison medical attendants have frequently acted as agents of social discipline and contributed to the policing of social divisions and the maintenance of order in individual institutions.

Health issues in prisons were closely associated with the development of prisons, and particularly their use as places to keep prisoners until ransom or execution, rather than as longer-term punishments in their own right. With the growth of prisons as a site for punishment through deprivation of liberty, health issues were probably exacerbated as facilities designed for relatively small numbers of inmates became more overcrowded. It was widely understood that due to health conditions in prisons, death or serious illness could be expected. This was largely due to their facilitation of infectious diseases such as typhus, scurvy, poor nutrition, and debilitating environment. With the almost simultaneous appreciation of the germ theory of disease, and the increasing use of close surveillance associated with the panopticon model of the prison (including solitary confinement), infectious disease morbidity and mortality in prisons began to decrease in the late 1800s. Nevertheless, even with the understanding of the action of infectious agents, prisons were and still are excellent sites for disease transmission. As in the law, context is everything: Pasteur himself noted that "the microbe is nothing, the terrain everything" (Crawford, 2007, p. 212). There remained, however, an often unstated understanding that the health risks of prison and specifically "lesser eligibility" were an integral part of the deterrent pains of imprisonment, notwithstanding the efforts of prison reformers such as John Howard, Elizabeth Fry and others.

3 Approaching health, law and human rights in prison

Comparing England and Wales and the European Court of Human Rights, and the United States

Despite having the benefit of emerging from a similar legal system, laws in the United States and England that deal with health-related rights of prisoners have diverged. The establishment of the US Constitution and the prohibition on cruel and unusual punishment has directed US approaches toward that test of whether a health care deficit or practice can be seen as a cruel or unusual punishment, an approach that has, however, come to be recently reflected in England since appeals to the European Court of Human Rights are, based on Article 3 of the European Convention on Human Rights, couched in similar language ("no-one shall be subject to torture or to inhuman or degrading treatment or punishment"). The wide differences in the content and amount of case law relating to health care in jails and prisons, however, would appear to be also based on contextual factors in the two jurisdictions. While it appears that prisoners are more litigious in the United States, this could be due to different approaches to legal funding (in the United States a successful litigant might expect to be awarded their fees, and lawyers may operate on the contingency of success). Further, the respective approaches to health care in the two jurisdictions are radically different, with the National Health Service (NHS) in the UK providing health care access for all, while the US system relies largely on purchased private or public health insurance, usually through one's employment, with differing safety-net entitlements on a state-by-state basis. While there is a view that health care is a right in the UK, in the United States it still tends to be seen as a service for payment rather than a right. The recent integration of the UK prison medical service into the NHS has emphasized the lack of conceptual difference between health care for those incarcerated and in the free world. In contrast, the United States is the "only wealthy, industrialized nation that does not ensure that all citizens have coverage" (National Institute of Medicine, 2004). Such differences in philosophical and funding approaches may also underlie the different volume and approach to prison health law in the two jurisdictions. Finally, there are different "filters" in the two countries which may partly account for the different volumes of cases. First, in the UK, the jurisdictions have officers – the Inspector-General of Prisons and the Health Ombudsman – whose position has been established specifically to deal with inadequate standards abuses in the prison system generally (in the case of the Inspector-General) and in health care specifically (in the case of the Health Ombudsman). There is also the post of Prison and Probation Ombudsman in the Prison Service in England and Wales, with specific staff positions for health matters. Thus, egregious or negligent practices are likely to be filtered out and dealt with before reaching the courts. Holders of the offices of Inspector-General of Prisons, Health Ombudsman and Prison and Probation Ombudsman have been extremely active (indeed, proactive) in defense of prisoners' rights. Second, there is also the cause of action of misfeasance in public office, alleging the office-holder has misused or abused their power, open to prisoners (which is not relevant here).

A European approach: England and Wales

The legal basis for the rights of prisoners while incarcerated, with specific implications for health-related rights, will differ across jurisdictions. In English law, the basis is summarized by Lord Wilberforce's judgment in *Raymond* v. *Honey* ([1982] 2 WLR 465), where he said: "Secondly, under English law, a convicted prisoner, in spite of his imprisonment, retains all civil rights which are not taken away expressly or by necessary implication." In order to understand what these rights that are taken away are, we need to examine subsequent case law.

The first principle of relevance is the prisoner's rights to suffer the minimum interference necessary. The relevant standards are set out first in the case of *R* v. *Secretary of State for the Home Department* ([1999] 3 WLR 328), where the prison authorities refused to allow continued visits of journalists unless the journalists signed undertakings not to use information obtained on prison visits for professional purposes, and the applicants – convicted prisoners – sought to overturn that refusal. The prison authorities argued that to allow any interviews by journalists would undermine proper control and discipline. The House of Lords held that while it was an inevitable consequence of imprisonment that a prisoner could not have an uncontrolled right to freedom of expression, any limitations "had to be justified by a pressing social need and as being the minimum interference necessary to achieve the objectives of deprivation of liberty by sentence of the court and discipline and order in prisons." Thus, an indiscriminate ban on journalistic interviews would infringe prisoners' right to seek access to justice. The applicants argued that unless there was a self-evident and pressing need for restrictions, and the measures adopted represented the minimum interference necessary to achieve the desired end, restrictions on prisoners' rights were outside the powers of the prison authorities. Legitimate objectives for limiting rights might be maintenance of secure custody, internal control and order and the prevention of crime. Countering this, it was argued that special weight should be given to prison administrators' experience and expertise in the area (a more conservative standard since prison administrators often tend to have more restrictive views of prisoners' rights).

In his judgment, Lord Steyn noted that the starting point is the assumption that the civil right is preserved unless it has been expressly removed or is an inevitable consequence of lawful detention in custody. In previous proceedings in this case in the Court of Appeal, it was argued by the prison authorities that there may be serious risk of distress to victims and their families. However, Lord Steyn noted that each particular case needed to be argued on its facts, and that the jurisprudence of the European Court of Human Rights had established that the term "necessary" as regards the words "necessary in a democratic society" requires the existence of a pressing social need, and that the restrictions should be no more than is proportionate to the legitimate aim pursued. In the case of prisoners' right to free speech, this right "is outweighed by deprivation of liberty by the sentence of a court, and the need for discipline and control in prisons." Lord Steyn raised the additional standard of what was consistent with order and discipline and administratively workable in prisons as being relevant to any limitation on civil rights of prisoners. Specifically, he noted that the principle of legality applies to subordinate legislation (such as prison rules and regulations) as much as to Acts of Parliament: prison regulations expressed in general language are also presumed to be subject to fundamental human rights. "Fundamental rights cannot be overridden by general or ambiguous words."

What constitutes "pressing social need"? In this case, "proper discipline and control includes consideration of the effect of inmates activities on others." Such others could include the victims of the crime, other inmates, staff and prison order and discipline. Prohibitions could be justified as part of a prison regime, but based on opinions of the European Court of Human Rights, in each case "it was necessary to carry out a balancing exercise but it concluded that a blanket prohibition was not necessary." The strong implication of the judgment in *R* v. *Secretary of State for the Home Department* is that the evidence must establish that a deprivation is necessary, based on prison order and discipline, the effects on others of the prisoner's activities, and that any restriction should not go beyond what is reasonably necessary. Thus, there is an onus on prison authorities to make the case on the evidence that a civil right should be restricted, and that blanket prohibitions are unacceptable.

The second principle of relevance is the restriction on rights and the "right-thinking members" of a democracy. Thus, on the other hand, a more recent English case (*R (on the application of Nilsen)* v. *Full Sutton Prison Governor* ([2005] 1WLR 1028)) which also involved freedom of expression (the applicant contesting the prison governor's decision to stop the applicant receiving from his solicitor a typescript of the prisoner's autobiography) takes a more restrictive view of civil rights in prison. In dismissing the applicant's appeal, the Court of Appeal noted that while it was not easy to define what the natural incidents of penal imprisonment were, "regard could be had to the expectations of right-thinking members of the democracy whose laws had deprived the prisoner of his liberty." It was noted that it was not disproportionate if imprisonment carried with it some restrictions on freedom of expression. It this case, the court determined that the prisoner's autobiography was not intended to "make serious representations about the safety of his conviction." It appears that the court more narrowly defined freedom of expression to refer to freedom to raise issues related to legal questions. The question here is who are the "right-thinking" in a democracy? Using the standard of what "right-thinking members of the democracy" might feel may not be appropriate given the fairly vindictive attitudes of some members of the public toward criminals and the high levels of emotion associated with crime and punishment. It is probably no more reasonable than asking right-thinking members of the public to determine appropriate standards of medical treatment for a particular disease. On the other hand, prison administrators might be considered the "experts" and have more conservative views on civil rights of prisoners than "right-thinking members of the democracy." More conservative views of prison administrators on prisoners' civil rights may understandably relate to the increased workload of providing additional or individual services in a system that is frequently understaffed, and to some prisoners insisting on additional rights as a way of asserting themselves or becoming obstructive in a system in which they have little power.

Standard of health care in prisons in the UK: the same for prisoners as for all people

Livingstone *et al.* (2008) summarize UK and EU law in regard to health issues. They note that the principles of medical ethics for prison staff follow those contained in the document adopted by the UN General Assembly in 1982 (UN Doc A/37/51), including the principle that treatment in prisons must be of the same quality and standard as is afforded to those who are not imprisoned or detained. From a European Community perspective, the Vienna World Conference on Human Rights of 1993 provides the same overarching principle: The prison system "must provide treatment to prisoners of the same quality and standard as is afforded to those who are not imprisoned or detained." This was confirmed in English law in *Brooks* v. *Home Office* ([1999] 2 FLR 33), where it was ruled that a pregnant woman was entitled to the same high standard of care whether or not she was serving a prison sentence. Note that this refers to a *high* standard of care entitlement: It might be thought that the Vienna Principle would allow for a low standard of care if that was what was available to those in the community, but the ruling in Brooks suggests that the prison health care standard should be set at the higher end of expectations. These principles include making it a contravention for any health personnel to participate in any procedure for restraining a prisoner or detainee unless for purely medical criteria. In England and Wales, health care in prisons has recently been transferred from the Health Care Service for Prisoners (formerly the Prison Medical Service) to NHS. This integration into the NHS ends the isolation of the prison health services from current developments in medical standards and training, and enables greater continuity of care between prison and community.

Internal prison standards

Prison service standing orders set out the legal position of the prison medical officer (every prison was required to have one up to 2007), including duties of examining prisoners for their first reception health screen within 24 hours of their reception, duties of certification as to fitness to work and placement under restraint. Prisoners' right to health care is protected by ensuring that every request by a prisoner to see a medical officer will be recorded by prison staff and passed on to the medical officer. Confidentiality of medical records is ensured, with the exception of cases where information received during a consultation indicates a clear threat to the safety of staff or other prisoners (*W* v. *Edgell* [1990] Ch. 359). The prisoner has a right to refuse treatment providing they can both comprehend and retain treatment information, and weigh it in the balance to arrive at a choice (Re C (Adult: Refusal of Treatment ([1994] 1 WLR 290))), even if that prisoner is compromised by reason of mental illness. Generally, a prisoner is held as being as capable as anyone else of giving consent to medical treatment. The Troubles in Northern Ireland also gave rise to questions on food and fluid refusal, and prisoners may not be forcibly fed or rehydrated while they remain capable of rational judgment, or if they have lost consciousness, whose families have not consented (*R* v. *Secretary of State ex parte* Robb ([1995] 1 All ER 677)).

The standard of health care in English and Welsh prisons is held to be that of the ordinary skilled health professional, using the skill of an ordinary competent person exercising that particular art. However, in *Knight* v. *Home Office* ([1990] 3 All ER 237), Pill J held that where a prison provided a lower level of staff to observe a suicide risk than would be available in a psychiatric hospital, that was not a breach of duty. His reasoning that the prison had a duty to safely detain, rather than a duty to cure, has been challenged by Livingstone *et al.* (2008), especially in the light of subsequent ECHR decisions that the state has a positive duty to take steps to protect life in situations of known risk. With regard to suicide risk, there have been several revisions of policy, and it was held in *Kirkham* v. *Chief Constable of Greater Manchester* ([1990] 3 All ER 246) that where a prisoner was identified as a suicide risk but this information was not passed on to prison staff, there is a breach of a duty of care to "take all reasonable steps to avoid acts or omissions which he could reasonably foresee would be likely to harm the person for which he is responsible." Livingstone *et al.*(2008) note that many suicides in prison would not have occurred outside, and arise from problems in coping with the experience of imprisonment. Given the heightened risk in prisons, assessment of suicide risk needs to occur, with a duty of care to avoid acts that could be reasonably foreseen would be likely to harm the person for which the prison is responsible. In *Orange* v. *Chief Constable of West Yorkshire* ([2002] QB 347), however, the court indicated that there were still risks that were unforeseen and unforeseeable. However, there is a move toward more active assessment of suicide risk rather than simply avoidance of acts and omissions that might create harm.

For mental health issues, particularly given the detention of a significant number of mentally disordered people in prisons, Livingstone *et al.* (2008) note that the standard of care must not be equivalent to a psychiatric hospital, but it must be a reasonable standard relative to the available resources. Health Care Standard 2 requires that a doctor who is psychiatrically qualified will have responsibility for the services, other health care workers will have had training in the field, all prisoners admitted to the prison health care unit will be seen within four hours and a present mental state assessment made. Where prisoners exhibit "challenging behavior" seclusion should be used as a last resort and medication should be prescribed only for clinical reasons. Overall, the English case law is less extensive than the US law, but this may be a function both of the existence of clear prison regulations with regard to health care of the incarcerated in England and Wales, and the lack of reliance on a standard of cruel and unusual punishment to regulate health care in prisons as in the United States. Livingstone *et al.* (2008, p. 300) observe that over 40 percent of prisoners in England and Wales have mental health needs, and many should not be in prison at all (but rather in a psychiatric facility or receiving treatment for mental disorders in the community).

Health-related rights (family life)

Health-related rights have been addressed in cases relating to the right of a prisoner who is married (in the absence of a policy allowing conjugal visits) to artificially inseminate his wife. In 2007, the European Court of Human Rights (*Dickson* v. *United Kingdom* [application no. 44362/04]) allowed the appeal of an English prisoner to provide for his wife's artificial insemination. The prisoner's wife would have been too old to bear children by the time of his release. The court made this ruling on the grounds of the right to family life and the right to found a family. It is consistent with an earlier US Court of Appeals case (*Gerber* v. *Hickman* (264 F.3d 882, 886 [9th Cir. 2001]), where it was found that this fundamental right to found a family "survives incarceration." These artificial insemination cases are important since the inability to associate with a conjugal partner is clearly a direct consequence of the inmate's limitation of freedom of movement and association by reason of deprivation of liberty. The health-related corollary, the right to artificial insemination where private conjugal visits are not permitted, provides for an alternate remedy. However, it also calls into question bans on conjugal visits, especially as they are allowed in a number of jurisdictions (Hopper, 1969) with no apparent detriment to order and discipline, and indeed with significant evidence suggesting that they substantially enhance order and discipline. In a related issue, that of the use of condoms in prisons, it was held that the decision should be made by the prison medical officer (presumably on medical and public health grounds). In *R* v. *Home Secretary ex parte Fielding* (1999), the court pointed out that on the condom issue, the inmate was "subject to scrutiny which would be unimaginable on the outside," suggesting that there may be areas of privacy relating to sexual behavior (sexual behavior between consenting adults of the same sex is not a crime in the UK or US) that may be applicable in prison as well as in the free world.

Other health-related rights: proper facilities, treatment, detoxification regimens

Not surprisingly, most cases relating to health-related issues in prison involve substance abuse and mental health treatment. In *McGlinchey* v. *United Kingdom* (2003), the European Court of Human Rights found that there were defects in health management and policy that constituted inhuman or degrading treatment. Ms McGlinchey was a heroin addict sentenced to prison who developed severe dehydration and weight loss from persistent vomiting, which subsequently led to her death. The defects the chamber noted included irregular administration of medication and inadequate medical monitoring which would have detected the seriousness of her condition prior to her collapse. The primary principle they found was that the absence of adequate requisite medical assistance amounted to distress or hardship exceeding the unavoidable level of suffering inherent in detention. Lack of adequate medical monitoring and assistance amounted, the chamber determined, to inhuman and degrading treatment. In another case also relating to a heroin addict in prison and withdrawing from the drug (*St George* v. *Home Office* [2008 EWCA Civ 1068]), Dyson LJ found the prison staff negligent in knowing about the prisoner's addiction and previous seizures, yet assigning him to a top bunk from which he fell, initiating *status epilepticus* and subsequently death. Dyson LJ noted that distinctions between actions that might be considered appropriate for such an individual in a drug rehabilitation clinic and in prison were spurious. Both share the common objective of weaning those in their care off drugs and alcohol and it is foreseeable to both that the person in their care may suffer a withdrawal seizure (or other effects of withdrawal). The second principle this opinion appears to establish is the need for common medical precautions regardless of whether the site is a clinic or correctional facility. That is, there is not a different standard of medical care or attention to medically related issues for prisons compared with equivalent non-custodial settings. Recent guidelines have been published (Department of Health, 2006) on the management of drug dependence in prison settings.

Further, where there is a serious mental disorder and the inmate is detained "without medical supervision appropriate to his current condition" and which entails "particularly acute hardship and causes distress or adversity of an intensity exceeding the unavoidable level of suffering inherent in detention" this is considered inhuman and degrading treatment (*Rivière* v. *France* [2006, application 33834/03, unpublished]). While this was a case where the prisoner was chronically psychotic and suicidal, the judgment appears to be sufficiently broadly worded as to encompass medical conditions beyond mental health cases. Recent ECHR cases have focused on the human dignity of the prisoner (in line with the "inhuman and degrading" standard): *Mouisel* v. *France* ([2004] 38 EHRR 34) was determined in part because the "treatment undermined his dignity and caused acute hardship over and above that inevitably entailed by his illness and the fact of imprisonment."

Finally, Livingstone *et al.* (2008) draw attention to the status of detainees in relation to asylum and deportation cases and the special health needs of such detainees, especially children and those who have been tortured. This is also an emerging issue in the United States, with large detention facilities serving asylum seekers, illegal immigrants, those detained awaiting immigration hearings and those awaiting deportation.

United States: health and human rights in prison

While US law is broadly based on the traditions of English law, the US Constitution forms the basis for most recognized rights. There is also much greater variability in legislation, with 51 legal codes (the 50 states and federal law) providing considerable variation. However, as federal law and the US Constitution supersede state law, there is an ultimate consistency in case law because on constitutional questions it has been appealed at a federal level. Like its English and European counterparts, human rights and health issues in the United States are based on the proscription of cruel and unusual punishment (Eighth Amendment). There is a large body of case law, perhaps due to the large prison population in the United States both in absolute numbers and per head of population; and perhaps due to the fact that the ideology of health access in the two countries is radically different. In the UK, since the foundation of the NHS in 1948, access to basic health care has been regarded as a right. In contrast, in the United States access to health care (with some states excepted) is largely based on a user-pays system, where health insurance (largely funded by employee and employer contributions) is the funder of health care.

Cruel and unusual punishment and the need for intent

The US Supreme Court decision that is the precedent for the standard for medical care in prisons is *Estelle* v. *Gamble* ([1976] 429 U.S. 97). *Estelle* v. *Gamble* noted the distinction between cruel and unusual punishment, as provided by the Eighth Amendment, and medical malpractice as recognizable in state courts. Marshall J notes that "denial of medical care may result in pain and suffering which no-one suggests would serve any penological purpose.... The infliction of such unnecessary suffering is inconsistent with contemporary standards of decency as manifested in modern legislation...." However, in the same judgment, Marshall J comments that "medical malpractice does not become a constitutional violation merely because the victim is a prisoner. ...a prisoner must allege acts or omissions sufficiently harmful to evidence deliberate indifference to medical needs." And, the acts or omissions which violate the Eighth Amendment are true "whether the indifference is manifested by prison doctors in their response to the prisoner's needs or by prison guards in intentionally denying or delaying access to medical care or intentionally interfering with the treatment once prescribed." In dissent, Stevens J notes:

> However, whether the constitutional standard has been violated should turn on the character of the punishment rather than the motivation of the individual who inflicted it. Whether the conditions ... were the product of design, negligence, or mere poverty, they were cruel and inhuman.

Estelle v. *Gamble* remains the standard against which Eighth Amendment claims relating to medical care in US prisons are assessed.

In the United States, Lindsley (2008) notes that while the state has the duty to make available to inmates a level of care that is reasonably designed to meet their routine and emergency health care needs (including physical, dental and psychiatric/psychological care), society does not expect that inmates will have unqualified access to health care. Where cruel and unusual punishment is concerned, there must be a demonstration of *deliberate* indifference to their medical needs, and *deliberate* withholding of care. Note particularly that the standard is cruel and unusual *punishment*, not poor health care, in this situation. Thus, the burden of proof is on the inmate to show that the health care or lack of care is being used as punishment, and the case law needs to be read with this in mind.

Lindsley (2008) states that delay in providing treatment (whether by prison guards or medical personnel) is actionable under civil rights statutes, but delay where the condition is not serious, not unreasonable or where no serious harm will result from the delay, does not state a claim. He suggests that the complaint must, as a minimum, allege all of the following: an acute physical condition; urgent need for medical care; failure or refusal to provide it; tangible residual injury; and "circumstances that will shock the judicial conscience." The delay needs to be intentional: in *Johnson* v. *Hamilton* (452 3d 967 [8th Cir. 2006]) a prisoner's claim was denied since there was no showing that the delay was the result of anything other than negligence!

Delay

Delay in diagnosis and treatment will not rise to the level of cruel and unusual punishment unless the delays are within physician control, and the delays can be demonstrated to contribute to the inmate's condition and are, importantly, *deliberately* indifferent. For example, a prisoner with only two lower teeth was not considered to have a serious medical need for dentures and so a dentist's delay of 15 months before providing dentures was not considered as violating the inmate's Eighth Amendment rights (*Farrow* v. *West*, 320 F. 3d 1235 [11th Cir. 2003]). Similarly, failure to schedule an optometrist's examination for four months was not considered deliberate indifference (*Wood* v. *Idaho Department of Corrections*, 391 F. Supp. 852 [D. Idaho 2005]). A 20-month delay in scheduling for surgery that was considered elective and where delay did not lead to a worsened prognosis was not considered detrimental to an inmate (*Buckley* v. *Correctional Medical Services, Inc.* (125 Fed Appx 98 [8th Cir. 2005]).

Prison staff serve as important gatekeepers for medical services, but are usually not medically trained. Thus, Lindsley notes, the official must know of and disregard an excessive risk to inmate health and safety, a state of mind that can be characterized as recklessness as used in criminal law (*Smith* v. *Carpenter*, 316 F. 3d 178 [2nd Cir. 2003]). Given the fact that prison staff are for all intents and purposes lay-persons in medical matters, the standard will be that of a reasonable lay-person. For example, it was held that severe heartburn and frequent vomiting from which a prisoner suffered was a "serious medical condition" from an objective viewpoint, since even a lay-person would have recognized the need for a physician's care to treat the condition (*Greeno* v. *Daley*, 414 F. 3d 645 [7th Cir. 2005]). However, in *Pizzuto* v. *County of Nassau*, 239 F. Supp 2d 301 [E.D. N.Y. 2003]), Lindsley notes: "Material issues of fact exist as to whether county corrections center supervisor knew that inmate had serious medical needs as a result of being beaten by two corrections officers, notwithstanding screams, moans, and other noises emanating from inmate's cell." The medical needs apparently have to be extremely obvious and serious. In *Jarriet* v. *Wilson* (414 F. 3d 634, F. App. [6th Cir. 2005]) the court held that a prison official must know of, and disregard, an excessive risk to inmate health and safety; the official must be aware of facts from which the inference could be drawn that a substantial risk of serious harm exists, and must also draw that inference. Those facts need to be obvious, and demonstrated to be obvious: Where a prison unit manager was shown not to be even aware that a prisoner had a serious medical condition and was suffering pain, because the manager had not taken the initiative to review the prisoner's medical notes over the course of a 13-month period, it was not held to be deliberate indifference in *Adsit* v. *Kaplan* (410 F. Supp. 2d 776 [W.D. Wis. 2006]).

Mere negligence

Medical negligence or malpractice in and of itself is not evidence of cruel and unusual punishment. Note, however, that medical or professional negligence may be actionable under other bases in civil law if serious injury results, or that it may give rise to complaints to state professional licensing boards regarding the professional competence or conduct of individual practitioners. This is not, however, a matter of civil rights and so not discussed further here. Differences of opinion between an inmate and health staff, or differences of opinion between medical staff, are not considered relevant to demonstrating a claim. However, where medical malpractice can rise to the level of deliberate indifference is where it involves culpable recklessness: An act or failure to act evinces a conscious disregard of a substantial risk of serious harm (*Atkins* v. *County of Orange* 372 F. Supp. 2d [S.D. N.Y. 2005]). Nevertheless, mental health medications in a "woefully inadequate dose" were not considered evidence of deliberate indifference, since the patient was seen and treated (even if inadequately medically: *Atkins* v. *County of Orange* 372 F. Supp. 2d [S.D. N.Y. 2005]). Other courts have held that even "serious negligence" or "gross negligence" are not sufficient for an Eighth or Fourteenth Amendment (deprivation of life, liberty or property without due process) claim. Deliberate indifference, the courts argued in *Cirilla* v. *Kankakee County Jail* (438 F. Supp. 2d 937 [C.D. Ill. 2006]), entails something more than mere negligence or even gross negligence; rather, deliberate indifference means that officials must want harm to come to the prisoner or at least must possess total unconcern for a prisoner's welfare in the face of serious risks. Thus, there must be a demonstrable state of mind on the part of the authorities to cause harm, and a serious risk that is so obvious as to be recognized by, depending on the target of the allegation, a lay-person, or by a medical attendant. Misdiagnosis and failure to conduct proper testing do not constitute deliberate indifference (*Self* v. *Crum*, 439 F. 3d 1227 [10th Cir. 2006]). A pharmacy providing incorrect medication to a prisoner is not deliberate indifference since there was no evidence of a culpable state of mind on the part of the pharmacy staff (*Davila* v. *Secure Pharmacy Plus*, 329 F. Supp. 2d 311 [D. Conn 2004]).

Where there is no medical difference of opinion, however, and the prison administration does not follow the therapy recommended, or denies it for unrelated reasons (such as the prisoner testing positive for illicit drugs), then this has been held to constitute "deliberate indifference." In *Johnson* v. *Wright* (234 F. Supp. 2d 352 [S.D. N.Y. 2002]) a prisoner was (despite unanimous opinion of his treating physicians to the contrary) denied Rebetron therapy to treat his Hepatitis C for 15 months because he tested positive for marijuana. Interference by prison authorities in recommended medical care where there is clear medical consensus does constitute a claim under the Eighth Amendment. On the other hand, *Martino* v. *Miller* (318 F. Supp. 2d 63 [W.D. N.Y. 2004]) did require a culpable state of mind and wanton intention to inflict pain to establish deliberate indifference for a violation of the Eighth Amendment based on medical care. Where a physician has prescribed therapy for a medical problem, and that therapy was denied on the grounds that the prison could not afford the treatment, this was held to state a claim for deliberate indifference (*Wilson* v. *Vanetta*, 291 F. Supp. 2d 811 [N.D. Ind. 2003]): The courts seem to generally regard overriding of medical treatment or prescription by non-medically trained staff as sufficient to establish deliberate indifference.

Mental health care is not considered distinct from other medical care for physical illness. Generally, Lindsley concludes, an inmate is entitled to treatment for serious psychiatric disease or injury provided it is curable or may be substantially alleviated, and that substantial harm will occur if care is delayed or denied. Unless there is clear evidence that delay in treatment adversely affects prognosis, there is no Eighth Amendment (cruel and unusual punishment) claim.

From the perspective of public health, delays in vaccinating for Hepatitis A and B did not violate the Eighth Amendment because despite the inmate's worry and distress, he did not actually contract Hepatitis A and B! There has to be evidence of specific harm arising from delay (to the individual making the claim) (*Wood* v. *Idaho Department of Corrections*, 391 F. Supp. 2d 852 [D. Idaho 2005]).

Environmental concerns

Environmental and safety issues in prisons, another area of public health interest, are covered by Lindsley (2008: §202, "Unhealthy, unsanitary, or unsafe conditions"). He observes that the government is due to exercise ordinary and reasonable care, under the circumstances, for preservation of an inmate's life and health. Again, deliberate indifference needs to be evidenced, toward a serious and apparent risk, for liability to exist. He further notes that there is no liability for mere inconvenient conditions and relatively minor hardships, or for minor or avoidable hazards. For example, unsanitary conditions that foster transmission of viruses and bacteria do not lead to a claim if the inmate cannot demonstrate that they or any other inmate actually contracted an illness through these unsanitary conditions (*Taggart* v. *MacDonald*, 131 Fed. Appx. 544 [9th Cir. 2005]). Further, there needs to be proof that the government agent being sued was deliberately indifferent to the conditions. In *Galloway* v. *Whetsel*, 124 Fed. Appx. 617 [10th Cir. 2005]) an Eighth Amendment violation was not established despite the fact that prison staff failed to provide the detainee with disinfectants and other appropriate supplies to clean feces from his cell floor and toilet, since it was not demonstrated that the county sheriff (the subject of the suit) was aware of the fact that staff had refused to supply the materials. Further, the death of an inmate from bacterial meningitis contracted in jail turned on the question as to whether the supervisory official had an *official* policy of maintaining the jail in dangerously overcrowded conditions and thus violated the inmate's Eighth Amendment rights.

Dietary and nutritional issues are central to public health concerns, given their implication in diabetes, obesity, heart disease, stroke, cancer prevention and many other public health issues. Nevertheless, dietary issues in prisons have not, except in extreme cases where clear and obvious medical outcomes occur, received support in case law. In *Baird* v. *Alameida* (407 F. Supp. 2d 1134 [C.D. Cal. 2005]) it was held that failing to implement policy to provide a "heart healthy" diet to inmates and failing to authorize therapeutic outpatient diets did not demonstrate that prison officials were deliberately indifferent to serious medical needs of an insulin-dependent diabetic. Despite his hospitalization for diabetic myelopathy while imprisoned, the court held that medical evidence indicated that the inmate's diet *could* be appropriate for diabetics, and the link between the diet and the inmate's medical problems was not proved.

Issues of environmental smoke have been similarly treated by courts. When an inmate with asthma was housed with smoking inmates for 17 weeks before being transferred to non-smoking housing, his Eighth Amendment suit was denied because there was no clear evidence that he needed any treatment beyond his existing inhaler. Further, even assuming serious medical need, there was no evidence of denial of medical care, or specific asthma attacks while housed with smokers. Thus, there was not considered to be a clear link *for this inmate at this time* between the smoky environment and specific medical harm. However, in *Bartlett* v. *Pearson* (406 F. Supp. 2d 626 [E.D. Va. 2005]) it was held that prison officials subjecting an inmate, with deliberate indifference, to levels of environmental tobacco smoke that posed an unreasonable risk of serious damage to the inmate's health, was cognizable under the Eighth Amendment and that showing aggravation of an existing medical condition was *not* required.

An example of the close linkage required for environmental conditions through to harm is provided in *Moody* v. *Kearney* (380 F. Supp. 2d 393 [D. Del. 2005]), where a state inmate alleged that he was on anticholinergic medication and particularly vulnerable to overheating and heat stroke; that prison officials knew about this vulnerability but acted with deliberate indifference by keeping him in a room with no windows, ventilation or access to running water when the temperature inside the facility was 120°F, and the inmate suffered severely debilitating heat stroke as a result.

Summary of US case law on health and constitutional rights

The neglect of poor or negligent health care for inmates in US law is not surprising, given that the vast majority of claims are based on the Eighth

Amendment which prohibits "cruel and unusual punishment." Thus, it is the issue of health care or its absence being used as punishment, not the quality of health care itself, which is central to an Eighth Amendment claim. Thus, the issue of intent to inflict harm is the crucial test, or acts or omissions sufficiently harmful to evidence severe indifference to serious medical needs – the *Estelle* v. *Gamble* criterion. Since there is no provision or right in the US Constitution regarding health care, cruel and unusual punishment is the most common vehicle for claims regarding health care. But the corollary is that health care issues such as negligence or substandard care are often secondary to the central claims under the Eighth Amendment (although less so to Fourteenth Amendment claims relating to death from poor or negligent health care in prison, as being deprivation of life without due process). It is not surprising that health rights do not figure specifically in the US Constitution. In 1787, at the time of the adoption of the Constitution, medicine could do little to alter the course of illness. There were few if any anesthetics (apart from alcohol), antiseptics, antibiotics or reliable medications, and disease was conceptualized as an imbalance of the four bodily "humors" (blood, yellow bile, black bile, phlegm). Treatments (such as bleeding a patient or applying leeches) were probably either largely ineffective or, in many cases, may even have hastened death. Thus, the concept that there was a "right" to health (since there was minimal if any control over health) would have, at the time, probably been regarded as fanciful. Consequently, human rights arguments relating to health care must use the closest vehicle in the Constitution, the prohibition of cruel and unusual punishment.

As will be noted from Lindsley's (2008) summaries of relevant US case law, health care in its provision or absence turns on its being considered as a cruel or unusual punishment. Foremost in the case law is the necessity to prove either intent, or such disregard of obvious risks that it is equivalent to intent. Second, case law is based upon individual requests for relief, and as such require a demonstration for that individual case. The chain of evidence from the health-related care or lack of care needs to lead logically and factually from this to serious harm to the individual: no harm, no punishment. There can be no dissent in the medical evidence or medical opinions, or else the presence or form of the treatment will be attributed to differences of opinion among professionals (or between professionals and inmates). Where the prison custodial staff act as gatekeepers to health care, as they usually do, the standard applied is that the health problem must be obvious to a reasonable lay-person. If a prison administrator is the subject of the claim, then there must be evidence that the problem was communicated through all the levels up to that administrator, or that the prison policy itself (and its specific application in the case itself) leads to the Eighth Amendment claim. Finally, since health care as such is not the issue in the Eighth Amendment, medical negligence or ineffective attempts to treat (absent demonstrated intent to use health care or its absence as punishment, or such a clear and obvious risk as to constitute deliberate indifference) are not accepted as the basis for a claim.

Conclusions

This review focuses on the constitutional basis for a finding of human rights violations: it must be emphasized that there may be other remedies for poor or negligent health care through other avenues of civil law, and complaints of professional negligence to state medical and nursing licensing bodies may be made where appropriate. Despite US law having its distant origins in English law, health rights in the United States and the UK have led to differences in both quantity and approach to cases on rights to health care, and the quality of that care. This may be due to two factors: first, the US health rights are based on a constitutional amendment relating to cruel and unusual punishment, and thus lack of care has to come up to that standard. In English law there is a specific set of prison regulations relating to health care, and so more directly health-related issues may be addressed directly as health issues. Second, the NHS in the UK has provided the whole population with a guarantee of basic health care, whereas in the United States there are vastly differing standards, ranging from high levels of care to almost none, and usually dependent on insurance funded from employment. These two factors may be partially responsible for the differences in approach and the different standards emerging from the two jurisdictions, with the US result appearing much harsher than that in the UK.

However, there are probably two major issues that influence the differences in approaches to prison health care rights in the US and English and Welsh systems. First, in the UK there is a filter system of the Health Services and Prison Ombudsmen, and the Inspector-General of Prisons, who are independent and proactive in promoting high standards in the prison system, and report independently to parliament. Second, in the United States the need to use constitutional provisions prohibiting cruel and unusual punishment as the vehicle for remedies to violations of rights in prison health care has led to lawyers trying to force the glass slipper of health onto the muscular foot of the Fourteenth Amendment. The result is the need to construct arguments relating to punishment rather than health. This combination of lack of any filter and the need to make inadequate health care fit a largely inappropriate standard appears to have led to the emergence of quite different bodies of case law in the United States and the UK. On the other hand, despite the differing approaches (cruel and unusual *versus* inhuman and degrading), there is nevertheless a degree of overlap between the two jurisdictions in the tests of what constitutes inappropriate care, with the standards of the typical practitioner or lay-person and judgment of level of indifference occurring in common. Nevertheless, the differing health philosophies and systems within which health care in prisons are embedded and the differing legal and financial climates for litigation from prisoners may also play some part in the issues that emerge into the light of case law in this area. The clear need for officials with jurisdiction to hear complaints, like the Inspectors of Prisons, or Health Ombudsmen, rather than to rely on tying complaints to constitutional provisions, may make for a more responsive approach to prison health standards in the United States.

4 The resurrection of the body in penology

Prison health care as physical punishment in a twentieth-century US correctional system

The notion of the body as a central concept in penology emerged with Foucault's (1977) thesis that the body as an object of punishment in public spectacles gave way in the eighteenth century to private punishment. This private punishment had a focus on the body as something to be organized and reformed, rather than subjected to pain. Foucault's thesis, however, skirts the possibility that despite the fact that formal sentences in western legal systems no longer include infliction of pain, informal sentences (those that are actually carried out in penal institutions) may include a focus on the body as a site of physical punishment and other disciplinary practices. If we are to examine the place of the body in late twentieth-century penology, prison medical systems and practices (where the focus is on the physical body) offer the opportunity to assess attitudes and practices that have the body as their target. Specifically, they may highlight the status of the body in prison. Is the sick body seen as an object for compassion or reformation (treatment) at one extreme (the medical perspective), or as an object for punishment at the other extreme (a punitive penological perspective)? Liebling with Arnold (2004, pp. 3–4) note that the late modern prison highlights the rapidly changing social context in which the prison currently exists, and the tension between this and the often outdated prison physical structure and experience (including health delivery). However, many late twentieth-century prisons, while exhibiting this tension, were not fully modern and thus I prefer the temporally situated term "late twentieth century." This tension might be exhibited both in prison disturbances and in court cases relating to prison conditions, and the treatment of the imprisoned body was frequently a focus of such action.

Foucault and the imprisoned body

In his treatise on the prison, Foucault (1977) suggests that there is a slackening hold on the body in modern prisons, in contrast to the public torture and capital punishment of malefactors before the late eighteenth century. He argues that the punishment–body relation is no longer what it was in the torture of public executions: "From being the art of unbearable sensations, punishment has become an economy of suspended rights" (p. 11). If the law manipulates the body, it will be at a distance, since the "body and pain are not the ultimate objects of its punitive action" (p. 11). Nevertheless, Foucault also notes that there remains in modern penal systems an element of torture, despite the progression toward more humanity (p. 16).

While Foucault may be correct, for western penal systems, that the public spectacle of the physical punishment of the body, with its public deterrence effect, is no longer in operation, the body has not disappeared from the penal system as he suggests (except for its disappearance from the formalities of the law). Brown (2009) argues that by "prison tourism," movies and other media, the imprisoned body does still remain as a public spectacle, albeit at a distance. However, it can be argued that the manipulation of the body in prison does not occur at a distance. The body may remain as the object of punishment in the prison system, either directly through informal brutality (which may in some contexts be sufficiently normative and institutionalized as to be semi-formal), or through health and illness in the prison, where the sick body may be the locus of additional disciplinary control. It is this second context that is the focus of this chapter.

Until the twentieth century, morbidity and mortality in prison from the effect of unsanitary conditions or infectious disease were high (Howard, 1784). However, the imprisoned body that is of most interest in the late twentieth and early twenty-first century is that of the inmate, where the health of the body (through provision of medically appropriate treatment, or through failure to prevent illness, failure to treat it or the use of inappropriate or punitive treatment explicitly as a punishment) marks the clear and unambiguous presence of the body in the penal system. Treatment as punishment is not a matter of pains inflicted on the body under law, but of informal intervention, and it is hidden precisely because it is in most jurisdictions *outside* the law. Thus, the body does figure significantly in the late twentieth-century prison, not just in terms of its temporal and spatial management, as Foucault describes, but in terms of being a site for punishment. In the twenty-first century, such bodily punishment (particularly in short-term facilities) may, however, be more rare.

Foucault has been criticized with regard to his approach to the body, knowledge and power in prisons. Garland (1990) argues that Foucault is imprecise as to the forms in which power was exercised, and the techniques and forms of power. This includes a failure to identify the agents of power, and what is designed to maximize control effects. He suggests (p. 163) that what is needed is to understand "the actual meaning-in-use" of power, and the limits on the type and extent of power. The body, Garland argues, may represent the individual's instinctive source of freedom, which resists and has to be dominated (p. 171). Of particular interest to the present chapter is his observation that a major source of resistance in prisons is alternative cultures (including inmate cultures). Such alternative cultures may develop their own language, identity and forms of conduct (p. 172). While Garland does not refer to medical cultures, this argument would certainly apply to medical culture, with its own well-developed norms, ethics, language, identity and perceptions of the individual at radical variance with that of the penal powers in the prison. It is an interesting question as to whether the threat of the development of a counter-penal medical "culture" or ideology may be one of the sources of the deprecation of the sick body as a locus for *medical* power, and the focus on the body as a site for the display of *penal* power. Supporting this interpretation, Sim (1990) notes how medical power (masquerading as knowledge), which defined the inmate as physically abnormal or mentally ill, was located firmly within the prison administrative culture, and within the Prison Health Service, largely isolated from mainstream medicine in the UK for the past century. It is possible that a vigorous assertion of the sick body as subject to penal, rather than medical, power may be an attempt to locate power over the body in the prison administration rather than in the alternative, and antithetical, power structure of medicine.

Subsequent to Foucault, Watson (1994) has noted that techniques of control and psychiatric knowledge appeared together as techniques to modify or reform the behavior of inmates rather than simply to punish them. Over-prescription and high doses of tranquilizing agents and other psychiatric medications may serve the purpose of modifying inmate behavior by sedation. Sim (1990) argues that prison medical services in the UK are part of a disciplinary web, but that its power has been contested both by prisoners and by prison officers. However, he suggests that while they may have some autonomy, prison medical personnel "did not stand outside or above the process" of disciplinary regulation, but were an integral part of it (p. 179). Watson observes that in the nineteenth and early twentieth centuries, there was a consolidation of medical power in prisons, and medical staff could modify or adapt penal regimes for special cases.

The body of the prisoner may also have enormous significance as an opportunity for expression. Brown (2009, p. 46) notes that prisoners are

> left with few avenues to engage in sociality beyond the use of their own bodies (the throwing of excrement, blood and urine; self-mutilation; suicide attempts). Of course, such behaviors are misconstrued by the penal spectator, who views such performance as pathology when, in fact, it is the starkest of socialities – the last line of an assertion of being and need for human relationships.

The "dirty protests" of IRA prisoners in Northern Ireland in the 1970s are perhaps one of the best-known examples. The use of the imprisoned body for self-expression in less negative or potentially more positive ways must also be acknowledged – for example, tattooing, body-building and an interest in health and fitness. However, the body of the prisoner as subject, rather than object, is beyond the scope of the present chapter.

As Foucault demonstrated his thesis through the historiography of cases such as Mettray and Neufchatel prisons as described in legal documents, I examine the thesis that the body remains a site for punishment in prisons through an examination of the *Ruiz* v. *Estelle* (503 F.Supp. 1265 [S.D. Tex. 1980]) case and its examination of the Texas prison system in the 1970s. *Ruiz*, like the historical examples of specific prisons selected by Foucault, offers ample legal documentation as a result of a long-running adversarial case and testimony under cross-examination. The Idar archive at the University of Texas also contains all the US press clippings on the case as it progressed, through to appeal and resolution. While I do not claim that the case is representative of all or even many of the large state prison systems in the 1970s (when Texas housed in excess of 20,000 prisoners), it does represent, in a large correctional system, a well-documented and debated example of the status and punishment of the body in late twentieth-century penology.

The Texas prison system in the context of the 1970s

Foucault (1977) suggests, following Rusche and Kirschheimer, that different systems of punishment are related to the systems of production within which they operate; for example, forced labor and the prison factory appear with the development of the mercantile economy. Carroll (1999) indicates that before *Ruiz*, "Texas prisons were run along the lines of old-style plantations" (p. 11). This comment is informative, and it might be instructive to consider the Texas prison system in the 1970s, the decade of the *Ruiz* trial, in this light. A full description of the origins and history of the Texas prison system is provided by Perkinson (2010). The late 1960s and 1970s were the decade of advances in civil rights, following the Civil Rights Act of 1964, and the political and social landscape of the US south was dominated by the issue. At the time, the racial/ethnic composition of the Texas Department of Corrections (TDC) inmates was 43 percent black, 19 percent Mexican ancestry and 39 percent white, the remainder being "other" (*Ruiz v. Estelle*, p. 22[1]). The vast majority of TDC officers at that time were white males from rural communities, with poor education and who received poor pay (p. 36). Further, the health care debates in *Ruiz* are often focused on work classifications and the ability of inmates to work in the fields (p. 64). The health issues often arose as inmates were classified for work which they could not perform for a variety of health- and medical-related reasons. Thus, tension over the body arose in part in the lack of correspondence between the needs and assumptions of the work classification system and the medical system. Some of the tensions leading to the *Ruiz* case might reasonably be seen as having arisen, at least in part, from the demographic characteristics of the inmate population and the TDC staff, the civil rights landscape and the longstanding history of East Texas as a plantation state and member of the Confederacy. That many of the health tensions arose over the classification of inmates and the health of their bodies relative to working in the fields or gardens may not be coincidental, and Carroll's (1999) analogy of Texas prisons as being run as old-style plantations (with the implication that elements of antebellum slavery continued) was probably pertinent.

The *Ruiz* v. *Estelle* case

Ruiz v. *Estelle* commenced in 1972 with a handwritten 15-page complaint by TDC inmate David Ruiz alleging violation of his constitutional rights, specifically Amendments 8 (prohibiting cruel and unusual punishment) and 14 (right to due process and equal protection) of the US Constitution, through prison overcrowding, deficient health care, unconstitutional supervision and security, including unlawful solitary confinement, unlawful discipline, unlawfully restricted access to the courts and other issues relating to confinement. The case was heard before Chief Judge William W. Justice of the US District Court for the Southern District of Texas and lasted over 161 days, over which 349 witnesses were called. Ruiz's complaint was joined with those of seven other inmates as a class action. In December 1980, the case concluded with a Special Master being appointed to closely supervise the TDC and bring about reform of the TDC system: Carroll (1999) has referred to the TDC pre-*Ruiz* as a "separate, isolated and largely autonomous moral order, almost immune to criticism and relatively untouched by evolving legal standards" (p. 11). The case was appealed and upheld by the US 5th Circuit Court of Appeals. For 15 months TDC Director Estelle and senior corrections officials defied the comprehensive and detailed judgment and remedial decrees, resigning only in 1983–1984. The conditions set by the court were largely satisfied in 1992, with the final issues resolved in 2002. Reynolds (2002) refers to *Ruiz* v. *Estelle* as the "most far-reaching prison conditions litigation in American history" (p. 1).

The *Ruiz* case decision was over 100 pages, with close attention being paid to one of the questions at issue, health care in TDC units. It thus provides a detailed description of health care-related conditions in a large US state prison system with a specificity, scope and richness of example that document and comprehensively describe prison conditions in one jurisdiction in the late twentieth century. As a historical document, it has the advantage of providing descriptions arising from nearly 350 witnesses for both sides, tested in cross-examination. Disadvantageously, it arises from a case alleging major deficits in the Texas prison system, and thus focuses on these failures and deficits in the system. It nevertheless provides an analyzable record of issues and themes in late twentieth-century prison health care, among other subjects, to allow an understanding of prison health care at this time and place. Specifically, it allows us to evaluate the status of the body and health in this context from inmate and staff perspectives. The court decision and press reporting of the case were read, extracting mentions of inmate illness, health and health care, and organizing these into themes and domains illustrating the TDC attitude and practice regarding inmate illness.

Unworthy of treatment, and health care neglect

The *Ruiz* case establishes that the body of the prisoner was not just unworthy of care, but that it was an additional occasion for penal sanction through neglect. This goes beyond what Sim (1990) refers to as "lesser eligibility" considerations, where the prisoner is regarded as having lower eligibility for health care. The issue of unworthiness for care was demonstrated by the low level of competence of health care workers in the TDC. The judgment (p. 55) describes the health personnel as often unqualified, wholly insufficient in numbers and deficiently supervised; and the meager medical facilities as inadequately equipped and poorly maintained. The medical care "system" (quotation marks in original) was marked by the absence of any organizational structure, plan or written procedures for delivery of medical care. To meet minimum American Correctional Association standards for the number of inmates, in 1974, 19 physicians needed to be employed; the TDC employed one. Even in May 1979, the system employed one physician for every 2,900 inmates (the ratio the US federal correctional system considered appropriate was 1:500).

The attitudes of health care personnel in the TDC came under strong criticism in the judgment, which referred to cases of "callous indifference on the part of physicians" (p. 56) and cited cases of refusing to treat, or treating and abandoning, seriously ill inmates. In fact, the core of the problems appears to be the use of lay personnel, "inmate helpers" or "medical assistants" to deliver treatment. This occurred to some extent because physicians, nurses and other professional health care workers found conditions intolerable and would not work in, or left, the TDC system. Those who remained were often unlicensed or unqualified for their positions (p. 56). Illustrating this, five registered nurses (RNs) and several licensed vocational nurses (LVNs) were employed at the Huntsville Unit Hospital (HUH, the central TDC infirmary) and "these nurses, who were apparently competent, well-trained and conscientious found conditions at HUH intolerable." After two years, all had resigned. One group resigned *en masse* and gave as their reasons the inadequacy of the physician staff, absence of any formal procedures and the TDC's lack of commitment to improving the level of care (p. 56). It seems that almost no professionally trained health workers were prepared to tolerate the conditions under which they had to perform, or the use of health care (or denial of care) as a form of punishment. The response of the TDC is telling in this regard: after the mass resignation of nurses, the TDC did not attempt to recruit more nurses, even minimally trained ones, but turned instead to medical assistants (MAs) to provide care. The judgment describes most MAs as "neither licensed, certified, or trained to accomplish auxiliary health care functions," yet they "routinely perform procedures that properly should be undertaken only by a registered nurse or a physician" (p. 57). The failure of the TDC to even attempt to employ RNs and LVNs demonstrated "its virtual abdication of responsibility for the provision of adequate health care for inmates" (p. 57).

This state of affairs is illustrative not only of the attitude of the TDC to health care at that time, but more specifically a likely intention to operate without licensed health care workers because appropriately trained health care workers would not accept the dominant punitive ethos surrounding health care. Health care workers at all levels are trained in ethics, standards of care, and imbued with the ethos of being a caring professional. After the mass resignation of nurses, it must have become apparent to the TDC that the problem was not solely one of working conditions and pay, but of diametrically conflicting standards: the sick body as being in need of care versus the sick body as an object for punishment. The solution was to employ MAs who were untrained in the ethos of care and indeed untrained in health care at all in many cases. MAs included inmate helpers and civilians who were imbued with the prevailing view of the inmate as not only unworthy of care, but worse, as manipulative malingerers or as objects for whom any opportunity for punishment should be taken (including in sickness). The judgment describes the health care system as being regulated by people only qualified to perform orderly functions and with "insensitive, casehardened sentiments" toward inmates (p. 58) and only available during daytime work hours. The judgment also notes that only one or two had medical-related licenses of any kind, and generally had no qualifications, no training and no supervision. They determined whether an inmate received any treatment at all, what medication to prescribe, when to request examination by a physician (if one were available) and when to refer to HUH or the Galveston hospital. They "conduct sick call, diagnose ailments, prescribe and dispense medicine, and watch over the health of inmates in solitary confinement" (p. 58). What we see here is not simply a move to replace health service professionals with untrained and unqualified staff, but more significantly, its replacement with staff who both lack the training to appreciate the unethical or negligent nature of "treatment" and also see the health system at the TDC as an extension of a function to punish and dehumanize the inmate. This was a health system *for* punishment and *as* punishment. Watson (1994) has described prison medical and psychiatric professionals as being likely to perceive themselves as protectors of the inmate rather than as the arm of the administration (p. 132). Removing such "protectors" and replacing them with personnel largely untrained in the health care field ensured that any potential protection of the inmate's body was removed.

To further show that the health system to be under the control of security staff, the judgment noted that "inmates form the backbone of the TDC medical system" (p. 58). The inmate in the health system, known as a "trusty," is the equivalent of the "building supervisor." He controls other inmates through violence or coercion on behalf of the (frequently heavily understaffed) security personnel. In addition to having no training, no supervision by qualified health personnel and being "deplorable obstacles to effective treatment" (p. 58), the *Ruiz* judgment notes that the inmate "nurses" (quotation marks added) had enormous authority over ill inmates (including the possibility of coercion, bribery [which was common] and extending violence to ill inmates). The "nurses" had a complete lack of understanding of confidentiality, but had access to confidential material that could be used to extort sexual or economic favors from other inmates. This was combined with "grievous neglect of the personal care of patients" (p. 60).

The judgment notes occasions that inmate "nurses" had been instructed or permitted to make deliberate falsifications and insert spurious readings in patient charts (p. 59). The evidence, according to the judgment, showed that inmate "nurses" X-ray and pin bone breaks, administer intravenous injections, perform Pap smears, prescribe and dispense drugs without the supervision of a physician or nurse, suture lacerations, conduct and interpret eye examinations, administer oral anesthesia, lance boils and insert catheters. There are extensive examples provided (p. 59) of mistakes in these areas made by inmate "nurses," who make medical errors which increase their patients' pain and suffering. Further, "grievous neglect of the personal care of patients" occurred (pp. 59–60): urine bags allowed to overflow; specimen collections not carried out or not refrigerated; intravenous solutions allowed to run dry; inmates allowed to lie in their own urine and feces for long periods; inadequate hygiene was administered; and bedsores were frequent in bed-ridden patients. Dental health followed the same pattern as medical care, with the judgment noting (p. 60) that inmates without training have been responsible for evaluating incoming inmate dental needs and that this "flagrantly improper practice" results in "extensive suffering for those inmates whose dental problems have not been properly diagnosed or treated." It is unclear whether this level of unqualified and largely negligent health care came about as a result of indifference, from a view of inmates as unworthy of decent health care, or from a deliberate attempt to enlist health care as part of a system of punishment. Regardless, the effect was to ensure that there was a seamless extension of the punitive regimen from the prison to the health system. The body of the inmate was an object of punishment, either in health or in illness through denial of treatment, or negligent treatment.

The Erewhon principle in prison health care

Seeing the sick body as subject to additional disciplinary control may constitute a specific assumption of health care in some correctional settings. The perception of health care in prison as being an integral part of the punitive environment, and indeed an integral part of the purpose of incarceration, forms what one might call the "Erewhon principle." *Erewhon* was the title of Samuel Butler's (1872) utopian but satirical novel, set in nineteenth-century New Zealand. In *Erewhon*, Butler stumbles on an advanced civilization where attitudes to sickness and crime have been reversed. Illness is treated as a crime, receiving widespread condemnation, and the ill are sentenced to punishment, including imprisonment, depending on the severity of their condition. In contrast, people who have committed crimes gain secondary sympathy and compassion from others. They are sent to "straighteners" (the Erewhonian equivalent of the medical profession) to be "cured":

> ... in that country if a man falls into ill health, or catches any disorder, or fails bodily in any way before he is seventy years old, he is tried before a jury of his countrymen, and if convicted is held up to public scorn and sentenced more or less severely as the case may be.... But if a man forges a check, or sets his house on fire, or robs with violence from the person, or does any other such things as are criminal in our own country, he is either taken to a hospital and most carefully tended at the public expense, or if he is in good circumstances, he lets it be known to all his friends that he is suffering from a severe fit of immorality.
>
> (1872, pp. 67–68)

The perception that the sick body is an additional and acceptable opportunity for disciplinary control parallels Butler's satire of sickness as subject to sanction or punishment. The apparent widespread practice of targeting the sick body illustrates that there is an underlying assumption (the "Erewhon principle") that sickness may, or should, be punishable. This can arise from the assumption that almost all prisoners are either malingering or exaggerating symptoms to gain sympathy or better conditions, or that they are at fault for their illness. The evidence in the *Ruiz* case is unclear as to whether it is the sickness *itself* or the sick *role* which elicits punishment, or whether it presents a better *target* for disciplinary practices.

Health care sabotage

Security and discipline concerns are a legitimate, indeed primary, concern of correctional environments, and in practice often take precedence over all other issues, including health care. They do not, however, from either a human rights or a medical perspective, take precedence over all other issues. Nevertheless, the perceived primacy of security and discipline concerns may also serve to legitimize the intrusion of punishment issues into health care. Such intrusion may be through discounting of health needs – "chilling indifference" to prisoners' health needs (p. 61) – or through active sabotage of treatment. Such active sabotage may occur under the guise of legitimate security issues such as the confiscation of prisoners' medications for verification on entry to a correctional facility. Such verification may take from hours to a week, during which time inmates are without medication. This results in "much unnecessary suffering" (*Ruiz*, p. 63) and is supposed to be circumvented for inmates with heart conditions, epilepsy or diabetes who are directed to notify Diagnostic Center officials immediately so that prescribed medication may be verified promptly. This change came about following the death of an inmate in 1974, whose anti-convulsant medication had been confiscated pending verification, but the court criticized this limited list of three conditions, noting that chronic conditions such as high blood pressure or asthma also need prompt attention (p. 63). The court also noted that despite the 1974 death, Diagnostic Center officials have since denied certain inmates necessary anti-seizure medicines pending absolute confirmation of their condition. Similarly, asthmatic inmates must surrender and be deprived of their medicines until a physical examination is conducted. Such a physical examination may take several days – even inmates with observable and potentially fatal conditions requiring immediate medical attention (e.g. gangrene) were forced to wait several days before receiving treatment (p. 63). The TDC argued that waiting for an inmate deprived of their medication to have a seizure, heart attack or asthma attack or to go into a diabetic coma would serve to provide accurate verification of the inmate's condition. The court noted that these practices resulted in "acute distress, discomfort and suffering by the affected inmates, and, moreover, carry with them a high potential of danger to the inmates". These practices are "dangerous in the extreme and cannot be justified as necessary for security" (p. 63). These practices may also be regarded as active sabotage of health.

A second practice that may be considered active sabotage of health is partly driven by the perception that most prisoners with medical problems are malingerers (p. 66). This hinders ongoing treatment. Frequently, warders and other prison officials ignored, cancelled or prematurely terminated lay-ins ordered by medical personnel, often with resultant serious complications or re-injury. Instances in *Ruiz* which make it clear that there is deliberate sabotage of medical orders include the following:

> An inmate was recovering from knee surgery and prison officials were directed to locate the inmate on the ground floor while at work, to avoid his having to climb stairs. Prison officials complied with this specific direction, but refused to move him from his cell four floors up, so that he had to climb three flights of stairs several times a day. They noted that the doctor's instructions referred only to the inmate's work assignment.
>
> (p. 65)

> An inmate with internal bleeding was sent back to his unit with an order not to do heavy lifting. Notwithstanding the physician's order, he was

directed to lift an oven on his return, resulting in his return to hospital with chest pain.

(p. 67)

After being treated for a complicated back problem, which included back surgery, an inmate returned to his unit with his doctor's instruction that he do no strenuous or heavy lifting for up to six months. He re-injured his back on a job assignment that required him to push bricks up a steel ramp.

(p. 67)

David Ruiz, the plaintiff in the case, was forced to work in the fields despite wearing a cast on his foot and barely being able to walk. In order to work, he had to remove the cast, even though his foot had not healed.

(p. 67)

An inmate recovering from hernia surgery had his medical lay-in cancelled by a medical assistant and was sent to work in the agricultural fields. This so traumatized the hernia repair that one of the inmate's testicles atrophied, and had to be surgically removed.

(p. 67)

These five examples indicate a degree of active sabotage of physicians' instructions by prison staff. Indeed, testimony by one physician indicated that "security personnel interfered with changes ordered by himself and other physicians, with the consequence that inmates remained in inappropriate jobs" (p. 67). The medical director indicated that instructions regarding treatment and work assignments could be made by physicians, but that they were ultimately at the pleasure of the warden. The court noted that "security personnel can and do interfere with the rehabilitation of inmates, and that Dr G [medical director] is apparently powerless to prevent it" (p. 88). Active sabotage of medical treatment appeared to be a routine practice in the TDC at that time.

Health care as punishment

There are also examples given in *Ruiz* of health care being administered in a punitive manner. Examples include lacerations being sutured without anesthesia as punishment, a catheterized patient going to empty his urine bag being ordered back to his cell, and when he protested, being attacked by security staff and having his catheter pulled out (p. 70), and over- or under-medication. Medical assistants wrote drug orders (despite being completely untrained in the area), and the judgment noted that many medications were diverted for their own use. A review of records indicated that about half of the patients had not received the medications prescribed for them, and psychoactive drugs such as Thorazine (chlorpromazine) were given at two times the maximum safe dose, with no observation (the drug is known to cause significant hypotension), in order to control inmates. The court noted that "The record is replete with countless examples of inmates who were subjected to incalculable discomfort and pain as a result of the lack of medical care or inadequacy in the treatment administered" (pp. 76–77). It continued with: "These examples fortify the conclusion that deficiencies were not isolated and bespeak of callous indifference to the welfare of inmate patients" (p. 77). They established "a continuous pattern of harmful, inadequate medical treatment which manifests itself frequently and injuriously in the lives of inmate-patients" (p. 77).

Punishment also occurred where inmates complained about the medical treatment or access to treatment. Disciplinary hearings (which the court noted invariably denied due process and which might be decided in a few seconds, and often included the officer who had made the complaint sitting in judgment) usually led to solitary confinement. Meals in solitary confinement contained only 10–16 percent of the recommended daily dietary allowances (p. 103) and were "drastically deficient in vitamins and minerals" (p. 106). Indeed, even previously healthy inmates suffered significant weight loss and when there were existing medical problems, the consequences could be extremely serious (p. 103). Time limits on solitary confinement were usually ignored. Despite TDC policy that diabetics were not to be put into solitary confinement, this happened; inmates would be removed from solitary confinement "semi-comatose" (p. 104). Medical checks on inmates in solitary confinement were performed by personnel who made observations of the inmates by only momentarily looking through the cell doors into the poorly lit cell (p. 104).

Health care as punishment assumes intentionality: specifically, the intention to make punishment permeate through all aspects of prison life. It should be differentiated from mere opportunistic brutality (what Brown [2009, p. 196] refers to as the "propensity to pounce on wounded or vulnerable individuals") which may be more of an individual rather than an institutional response. However, routinely taking the opportunity of attacking a sick individual when they are at their most vulnerable rises to the level of an institutional abuse of the sick, given its pervasiveness in the TDC system at that time. In *Ruiz* the court makes it clear that the prison health system (or lack of one) was pervaded by an ethos of penality.

Potemkin infirmaries

The health system as described in *Ruiz* amounts to a Potemkin village system – one which is maintained to give a show of health care while covering up the reality of abuse and misery. The term arises from "Potemkin villages," named for Prince Grigory Potemkin, the prime minister of Catherine the

Great of Russia in the eighteenth century. Potemkin had fake village façades, populated with actors who played happy and prosperous villagers, erected along the route of the empress. After she had passed, the villages and actors were packed up like Hollywood sets and redeployed ahead of her progress to give her the impression that her subjects were content and flourishing, while the real poverty-stricken villagers were kept out of sight by the troops until she had passed. The TDC health care system described in *Ruiz* amounted to little more than a façade to hide the lack of qualified health care staff, and to replace them with agents of a system that apparently regarded health issues as simply another opportunity to punish the inmate by acts of omission or commission. MAs and inmate "nurses" appear to have been preferred because they were not imbued with a protective medical or health care culture, but were instilled with the prevalent punitive prison culture. At its worst, such a system could be actively set up to promote malpractice, give an appearance of appropriate health care and promote indifferent, negligent treatment or deliberately avoid treatment. Further, where medical treatment was prescribed, the prison system may have actively sabotaged that treatment. The body, far from being removed from the realm of punishment, as Foucault suggests, remained a focus. This focus, however, was opportunistic, upon the occasion of illness, rather than deliberately inflicted as a formal punishment by courts.

The "Potemkin infirmaries" and the poor conditions raise a further Foucauldian theme, that of architecture and function in prisons. The poor physical conditions and lack of facilities and equipment suggest that Texas prisons were designed with little or no health care in mind, and the lack of facilities and poor fabric in the Huntsville "prison hospital" reinforce this by the fact that there had been almost no attempt to provide or update equipment or services. The combination of pitiful facilities and the "Potemkin" nature of the "improvements" support the view that health care was not intended in the prison system. This view re-emerges in the subsequent consideration of the lack of adequate health facilities in the California correctional system (*Plata/Coleman* v. *Schwarzenegger* [2009] – No. CIV S-90-0520 LKK JFM P 2009, WL 2430820 [E.D. Cal. Aug 4, 2009] combined with *Plata* v. *Schwarzenegger* No. C01-1351 THE, 2005 WL 2932253 [N.D. Cal. Oct 3, 2005]).

Prison physical and social climate

In *Ruiz* v. *Estelle*, the Court made extensive note of the deficient physical plant associated with health. Occupational health and safety issues including fire safety, sanitation, overcrowding, food processing, and dangerous and unsafe inmate work conditions were all described as contributing to potential or actual health and safety risks (p. 115). The HUH, the main prison hospital/infirmary, was described as "Antiquated, poorly designed, unacceptably equipped, and deficiently maintained" (p. 61).

The court commented (p. 46) on the widespread culture of prison brutality (pp. 46–54). In the section of the *Ruiz* judgment on staff brutality it is noted that the record is replete with credible evidence of inmates being unreasonably and unmercifully beaten with fists and clubs, and kicked and maced by officers, with many of the injuries inflicted requiring medical attention. They noted that "brutality against inmates is nothing short of routine in the Texas prisons" (p. 46) and that there were "numerous incidents of needless, savage physical brutality against inmates who were already subdued or who had not participated in whatever confrontation had occurred." It seems reasonable to assume that the brutality which led to the injuries suffered by inmates was continuous with subsequent indifference to unnecessary suffering during, or brutality of medical care of such injuries. The evidence in *Ruiz* consistently points to the fact that health and medical issues do not, by their appearance, engender different and compassionate approaches to inmates on the part of prison staff. The view of the inmate in sickness and in health does not change: those who are by their status as inmates dehumanized in one context are dehumanized in all other contexts, with the rationalization that any symptoms of sickness are largely "trickitis" (malingering) (p. 68). Indeed, far from the ill being seen as deserving pity, the illness was seen as a further opportunity for staff to exercise power and use it as an occasion for active (malpractice or punitive treatment) or passive (denial of treatment) punishment. In short, illness was not privileged in the Texas prison system as it was in the free world: it was simply another context in which the inmate could be brutalized or punished. Climate in the general (non-health) prison environment and climate in prison health care are components of the same system, and of the same staff attitudes and beliefs toward inmates and imprisonment. The interrelated nature of the various constitutional violations in *Ruiz* – overcrowding, security and supervision, health care delivery, discipline and denial or obstruction of access to the courts at the TDC (p. 124) – were all facets of the same climate. They formed, as the judgment noted, an aggregate, with the harms formed by each, in a legal sense, exacerbating the others.

The data from *Ruiz* raise the issue of prison climate as a *determinant* of prison health care. Liebling with Arnold (2004) argue that values are central to prisons, which they call "special moral places.... Places where relationships, and the treatment of one party by another, really matter" (p. xviii). Following Rutherford, they note three working credos of criminal justice (punishment – punitive degradation of offenders; efficiency — pragmatic managerialism; and care – humane containment) which describe the major values associated with the late twentieth-century prison (p. 7). These constitute major ideological dimensions which may steer prison performances in general, and staff conduct in particular. To the extent that a prison administration's values are punitive, then that will permeate all activities in the prison. It is difficult to separate out penal practices within a system or institution that, as Brown (2009, p. 31) observes, is a "complex overlapping and spiraling environment."

Access to health care in prison

Additionally, the issue of prison climate is also crucial not only where health care as punishment is seen, but also in terms of access to health care. In *Ruiz*, the mechanism to access care was the Sick Call. Inmates needed to request permission in writing the previous night to attend: building tenders and prison staff frequently refused to honor requests, or the inmate might be punished if the complaint was not considered to be substantive (p. 66). The inmate's access was blocked by untrained (in health care) security or inmate personnel. The system of requiring written notice to be given more than 12 hours ahead of Sick Call did not take into account emergencies, situations where the inmate was confused or in pain, or conditions that did not have sufficiently obvious signs and symptoms to persuade the building tender or security staff that the illness was genuine. Indeed, it appears that all illnesses were regarded as malingering unless there was clear and unambiguous evidence to the contrary. Thus, prison climate impacts all levels of health care, from initial access through to the level of health care provided, treatment and recovery or rehabilitation. Prison health care is suffused with the ambient prison climate, and its players – security staff, inmates, health care personnel, administrators – all acting and living within that climate.

One of the corollaries of prison health care is that by being embedded in a prison climate, in a relatively closed physical and social environment, the values and ethics of health care are overwhelmed by the values and ethics of the prison and its security. Ross *et al.* (2011) demonstrated that prison health care in the English and Welsh system was closely related to prison climate. They found that the prison social climate dimensions of relationships with staff, safety, level of feedback and care, fairness, and care for the vulnerable, were all associated with prison health care. They note in their qualitative interviews that introducing health care values into a prison system may overwhelm health care values and transform the health worker's values into the values of the prison system. ("we had hoped that bringing a whole lot of nurses in would infuse a nursing culture into our health care, but what we've found is that we have infused a prison culture into our nurses"). This is entirely consistent with the predictions of social psychology regarding adherence to a dominant or in-group's point of view. In prison, health care climates are essentially moral climates – the view that the inmate is in prison for punishment, in health matters a malingerer, and has forfeited his or her rights to be regarded as fully human at one climatic extreme, and the view that every person has a right to decent health care, regardless of their personal failings, at the other. The court in *Ruiz* (p. 123) moved toward the latter view: "No effort to punish inmates justifies exposing them to unnecessary health risks, for their confinement constitutes punishment enough."

Press coverage of *Ruiz* v. *Estelle*

The question arises as to whether the TDC system was an aberration in the Texas political and social context, or whether it accurately reflected a wider community set of attitudes with regard to treatment of inmates. A complete file of press clippings relating to the *Ruiz* trial and appeals was deposited two decades later in the University of Texas archives by Eduardo Idar, one of the attorneys representing the State of Texas at the trial, and casts some light on the community response.

Media reaction to the trial in the press was generally objective and recognized both the need for change and the extraordinary level of change the judgment proposed. The mainstream *Houston Chronicle* summarized the tension in this debate well when it referred to Judge Justice as a "devil-saint Federal judge" (Franks, 1981). The conflicted approach in the Texas press had earlier been summed up in the *Houston Chronicle* (Hunter, 1980) by acknowledging the feelings of shock conveyed by some of the testimony on prison standards as "trying to convey the impossible to convey" and in the same article noting that the judge applied no new legal standards but was "trying to force nationwide acceptance of unrealistic Federal prison standards in effect in other states." The *Huntsville Item* (Huntsville is the town in central Texas which contains the Texas Department of Criminal Justice [TDCJ, the current incarnation of TDC] headquarters and houses four prisons, the execution chamber, the TDCJ warehouse and prison store, the TDCJ medical unit, and where the TDCJ is one of the largest employers) was more sharply critical, with the comment that the ruling was "more a philosophy on how a prison system should be run rather than a valid analysis of whether or not TDC is depriving inmates of their constitutional rights" (Trow, 1980). In the appeal case, the *Huntsville Item* focused on apparent inappropriate procedures at the trial on the part of Judge Justice (headline: "Justice's procedures blasted," *Huntsville Item*, 1981). The more liberal (or perhaps more federal) *Washington Post* talked of the "wrenching description of life in Texas prisons" (Balz, 1981), while in 1981 the *Houston Chronicle* headlined "Deaths attributed to poor care in hospital in Huntsville prison" and "State finds TDC hospital staff to be unqualified," noting "serious shortcomings" and "medical mismanagement." Sympathy for the *sick* in prison, however, did not necessarily extend into sympathy for *prisoners*. The *Houston Chronicle* (1982) observed that the "court ... [was] choosing to believe all prisoners told the truth and that all prison officials lied."

A significant amount of disapproval was based on the fact that the federal justice system was seen to be interfering in the State of Texas: Governor Clements is quoted in the *Houston Post* as believing that the "[US] justice department should never have been in the suit in the first place ... our prison system is Texas state business and we think we know how to run a prison system" (West, 1981). Subsequently, a more nuanced approach to the issue developed, with the *Houston Chronicle* (Byers, 1982) noting that it was simplistic to blame the prison crisis on overcrowding (headline: "Wrong way to handle prison crisis"), and that "continuing to build maximum security prisons to house an ever-increasing number of inmates may be the worst foolishness of all. Texas needs to rethink the goals of criminal justice and what road to follow to achieve the goals." Simultaneously, the *Houston Post* (Vara, 1982) headlined that "TDC must face up to questions the crisis raised."

Not all opinion was so nuanced: support for pervasive punitive prison conditions (including health care) was also expressed. The magazine *Texas Monthly* (Reavis, 1985) acknowledged that Texas prisons were "places where, in defiance of the law, prisoners were punished by assault, by kicks and blows from guards and their convict allies, the building tenders ... wasting away on a diet of bread and water." He goes on to argue:

> However ugly, the system did most of the things we can realistically expect a prison system to do. It did them well, and it did them cheaply. Before the trial of *Ruiz v. Estelle*, prisons in Texas were the safest, most productive, and most economical in the nation. Today, they are the most dangerous.

The utilitarian argument was that the system "worked," and that "The answer to the Texas prison crisis is to run the jails the same way as we did 20 years ago" (Reavis, 1985).

The press and some facets of public opinion, however, did not always agree. When Judge Justice died in 2009, the *Houston Chronicle* editorial argued that he was "a genuine change agent in a state whose traditional ways of dealing with minorities and prisoners needed changing ... [he] transformed Texas, often kicking and screaming, and we are the better for his service." In an online comment on that editorial the same day, "Rancher" said "We did not need our jails improved. They needed to be a hellhole to be effective on the type of people we sent there." The media debate over the course of the trial and appeals reflects both a sense that the prison system was over-reaching in its targeting of the prisoner (and the sick body in prison), and a contrasting community perception that such punitive targeting was consistent with the mission of Texas prisons.

Policy implications

This analysis of *Ruiz* v. *Estelle* has several policy implications. If medical care in prisons is to become an additional occasion for punishment of the body, then medical care needs to be sourced away from the prison environment so that medical attendants are not socialized into prison values. This option has been addressed in the UK by Ramsbotham (1996), who observes that the range of problems faced by medical staff in establishments differs "only in degree" from those occurring in the rest of the community

(Foreword). Ramsbotham argues cogently that all prisoners requiring health care must be seen as patients and given the same care as provided in the community (p. 4). He notes that prisoners were members of the wider community before their reception into prison and the vast majority will return to that community on their release. Ramsbotham goes on to observe (p. 7) that it is illogical that just because they are prisoners, their health care is provided through separate channels, and that "It is also necessary to recognize the interdependence of health care in prisons and wider health care." This reasoning led to the transfer of prison medical services to the National Health Service (NHS) in the UK (Joint Prison Service and National Health Service Executive Working Group, 1999; Commission for Health care Audit and Inspection and HM Inspectorate of Prisons, 2009).

However, siting medical services outside of a prison may also lead to delays in treatment of emergencies if their location is too distant. While transfer of prison medical services to the NHS in the UK is a sensible option, in US states where there is no universal health service, and where 95 percent of prisoners are medically uninsured, this is not feasible. Contracting out medical services to a local medical practice may occur with more isolated, or private, facilities. Recently, the growth and extension of telemedicine for surgical, internal medicine and psychiatric consultations (e.g., Ellis *et al.*, 2006; Tucker *et al.*, 2006) has shown that real-time videoconferencing has considerable benefits for provision of high-quality medical services in prisons, and may even be preferred for prisoners with safety and sexual issues. While this does not necessarily deal with access to treatment and implementation of treatment issues, it does ensure an external medical gaze into the prison.

Déjà vu, California 2009: *Coleman/Plata* v. *Schwarzenegger*

In 2009, a case with some similarities to *Ruiz* was decided in California. The cases of *Coleman* v. *Schwarzenegger* and *Plata* v. *Schwarzenegger* were joined in the Eastern Federal Court of California as the culmination (subject to a Supreme Court appeal) of a two-decade-long battle over medical and mental health care conditions in California state prisons. The court ordered California to release between 37,000 and 58,000 prisoners to reduce prison overcrowding to the point where delivery of medical and mental health care to constitutional standards was possible. Prison overcrowding in California in 2009 was estimated at 190 percent and the court set 130–145 percent as the acceptable overcrowding range. Some of the 33 Californian institutions have populations approaching 300 percent of intended capacity. *Coleman* was filed in 1990 and *Plata* in 2001 (*Harvard Law Review*, 2010). The court found in *Coleman/Plata* that

> California inmates have long been denied that minimal level of [constitutional] medical and mental health care, with consequences that

have been serious, and often fatal. Inmates are forced to wait months or years for medically necessary appointments and examinations, and many receive inadequate medical care in substandard facilities that lack the medical equipment required to conduct routine examinations or afford essential medical treatment. Seriously mentally ill inmates languish in horrific conditions without access to necessary mental health care, raising the acuity of mental illness throughout the system and increasing the risk of inmate suicide. A significant number of inmates have died as a result of the state's failure to provide constitutionally adequate medical care. As of mid-2005, a California inmate was dying needlessly *every six or seven days*.

> (*Coleman/Plata*, 2009, p. 6–7; emphasis in original)

In *Coleman/Plata*, the court listed the deficiencies as: inadequate medical screening of incoming prisoners; delays or failure to provide access to medical care, including specialist care; untimely responses to medical emergencies; the interference of custodial staff with the provision of medical care; the failure to recruit and train sufficient numbers of competent medical staff; disorganized and incomplete medical records; a "lack of quality control procedures, including lack of physician peer review, quality assurance, and death reviews"; a lack of protocols to deal with chronic illness, including diabetes, heart disease, Hepatitis and HIV; and the failure of the administrative grievance system to provide timely or adequate responses to complaints concerning medical care (p. 11).

There are both similarities and differences with *Ruiz* and the argument that the body remained a site for punishment in prison. The similarity occurs in the accusations of custodial staff interfering with medical care, delay or denial or treatment, and minimal and sometimes incompetent medical and nursing staff and an almost complete lack of appropriate facilities.

The difference lies in the fact that the California system was grossly overcrowded, and that with the exceptions noted above, there was indifference on the part of the legislature and the administration to prisoners generally and by extension to their physical and mental health needs. This difference leads to prisoners *as a class* being subject to medical neglect and indifference in *Coleman/Plata*, whereas in *Ruiz* the evidence suggested that targeting the body of the sick inmate was a deliberate choice. In *Coleman/Plata* the evidence suggests that the devaluing of the body of the prisoner is a function of overcrowding and indifference rather than a specific intentional outcome. Notwithstanding this, the California court noted "multiple instances of incompetence, indifference, cruelty, and neglect .... most deaths were preventable" (p. 14); and death reviews revealed "repeated gross departures from even minimal standards of care" (p. 18).

The California and Texas prison systems are not only the largest state systems in the United States, but also among the largest in the world. The *Coleman/Plata* v. *Schwarzenegger* (2009) case is entirely consistent with

Ruiz, despite being decided nearly 30 years later, in demonstrating the potential for the punishment of the body of the sick inmate through neglect, indifference and medical incompetence. As with *Ruiz*, in California the body of the prisoner appears to be seen as having "lesser eligibility" – unworthy of treatment, and as worthy of neglect. *Coleman/Plata* also suggests, however, that specific targeting of the sick inmate for bodily punishment may be less apparent and hopefully less common (although *Coleman/Plata* did not turn, and thus evidence did not focus, on this point, but on the role of *overcrowding* in the inadequate provision of care). The US Supreme Court upheld the decision of the lower court in May 2011 (*Brown* v. *Plata*, 563 U.S. [2011]). Specifically, they noted that the overcrowding was exacerbated by high vacancy rates for medical and mental health professionals, difficulty in attracting well-qualified professionals and insufficient treatment space even if the positions were to be filled. The effect of the continuing injury and harm resulting from the "grossly inadequate provision of medical and mental health care" (p. 4) is a constitutional violation and "needless suffering and death have been the well-documented result" (p. 3). These include substantially increased risks for infectious disease transmission and unacceptably high suicide rates. Indeed, the court cited the former head of corrections in Texas as describing conditions in California prisons as "appalling, inhumane and unacceptable" (p. 5)! Consequently, the court set the overcrowding cap at 137.5 percent of capacity and affirmed that lack of medical and mental health treatment of the ill inmate, and conditions that create illness and exacerbate poor mental health, constitute cruel and unusual punishment and thus violate the Eighth Amendment of the US Constitution. The US Supreme Court effectively held that by ignoring or inadequately treating existing illness, and creating new illness, prisons are, in effect, imposing cruel and unusual punishment on the body of the sick inmate and creating new illnesses. What is particularly interesting is that in this judgment they found a *generalized* punishment of the body for a *class of persons* (inmates) as well as specific individuals, to be cruel and unusual punishment.

Conclusions

Analysis of *Ruiz* v. *Estelle* strongly suggests that, in the late twentieth century, there were jurisdictions where the body was an object of punishment, within a prison health system that was staffed and operated in such a way as to facilitate health care as punishment. Despite Foucault's (1977) contention that the body no longer figures in punishment, his position appears to relate specifically to the body in *formal* (by which I mean legally sanctioned) punishment. *Ruiz*, however, establishes that the body may still have figured largely in *informal* punishment. It is opportunistic – that is, the sick body is usually used as an occasion for punishment when the inmate is ill. Nevertheless, *Ruiz* does provide instances where inmates were injured by security personnel or "trusties" and health care was also denied. In this context, Foucault is correct in his analysis of the relations between prisons and power, and in *Ruiz* we see the prison staff as an alternative power, or as a lens through which power is distorted, ignoring the rulings, letter and spirit of the law.

Here, Foucault's concept of gaze is useful. The issue in *Ruiz* with regard to the informal punishments might be seen as a lack, or failure, of gaze. *Lack of gaze* created a blind spot in the monitoring of the prisoner, and rendered unavailable the potential remedies in a formal system such as appeal and review. Literally, justice was blind (and blinded) as to the operation of such an informal punitive system. The informal punitive system, being out of sight, permitted the punishment of the body which has long been removed from formal sentencing in western legal systems. Evidence from *Ruiz* suggests that lack of gaze from legal and medical authorities effectively allowed the TDC, in the 1970s, to maintain punishment of the body through the avenues of staff or staff-sanctioned brutality, and system- and staff-sanctioned use of the health system as another avenue for punishment.

A prison climate which sees the inmate as unworthy of humane treatment, and in prison *for* punishment, will engage in that punishment where the opportunity arises – in staff brutality toward the well and the sick, and in using opportunities as they arise to punish the body. For the sick body, restriction or denial of access to treatment, untrained staff who share the view that the inmate's body is an object for punishment or that most inmates are malingerers, painful or inappropriate treatment, or sabotage or denial of treatment, are largely opportunistic. A prison climate with a punitive view of inmates will attack their rights and their bodies with equal enthusiasm, precisely because they are seen as worthy of continuing punishment in the prison environment. That is, the body is there for punishment, and it is the role of the staff to provide it, in sickness and in health. Where there is lack of gaze to enforce law, health and safety and medical care (indeed, the word "care" in relation to prison health care in *Ruiz* is an oxymoron) will be determined by the ambient prison climate – and not by any considerations about health care as a special case or as an exception.

An examination of *Ruiz* v. *Estelle* (1980) provides a case history of a late twentieth-century western prison system where it is possible, given the level of detail of the evidence presented at the trial, to describe the state of the body in health care in a large prison system at that time. This legal record combines TDC statistics, site inspections and testimony of inmates, administrators, security staff, health personnel, former staff and expert witnesses, with testimony subject to cross-examination. It is apparent that the inmate body in this system was not only subject to punishment, but also that no distinction was made between the sick and the well. This was often rationalized by the view that the majority of inmates complaining of illness were malingerers and thus not really "sick." The free world view that the ill are entitled to care has no traction in the prison: sickness simply becomes another opportunity to punish the body of the inmate in a more varied and wide-ranging form. This could include denial of access to care, negligent care, punitive care, sabotage of professionally prescribed care, and its facilitation by setting up a health care system largely staffed by untrained and often inmate attendants who were imbued with the prison culture. *Ruiz* confirms the thesis that the body remained the object of punishment in at least one late twentieth-century western prison system, and particularly in a health context where the body, traditionally the subject of care, becomes the object of the infliction of pain and suffering. However, it would probably be a mistake to assume that the TDC was very different from most US state prison systems in the 1970s: it was simply the most extensively documented case due to the *Ruiz* trial. We can conclude that for health care, as Sim (1990) observed in an English context, violence retained a central place in the repertoire of responses mobilized by the state inside prisons, and that medical personnel did not stand outside or above the disciplinary process, but become an integral part of it (p. 179). *Ruiz* helps make the case that the body remained as an important, but under-recognized, concept in the late twentieth-century prison, at least in terms of prison health care and its subjection to the values and climate of the institution.

Notwithstanding *Coleman/Plata*, the argument arising from *Ruiz*, that the sick body was (and may still be) a major site of punishment, still stands demonstrated in the historical case of the Texas prison system in the United States in the twentieth century. *Coleman/Plata* simply reinforces the continuing potential for this to occur through neglect (rather than specific targeting) at a system-wide level into the twenty-first century. It may be that the inmate body in prison, and explanations for its treatment, remain a significant topic of investigation into the twenty-first century.

5 On giving good care to bad people

Examining the principles of prison health care

> The mood and temper of the public in regard to the treatment of crime and criminals is one of the most unfailing tests of the civilization of any country. A calm and dispassionate recognition of the rights of the accused against the State, and even of convicted criminals against the State, a constant heart-searching by all charged with the duty of punishment, a desire and eagerness to rehabilitate in the world of industry all those who have paid their dues in the hard coinage of punishment, tireless efforts towards the discovery of curative and regenerating processes, and an unfaltering faith that there is a treasure, if you can only find it, in the heart of every man – these are the symbols which in the treatment of crime and criminals mark and measure the stored-up strength of a nation, and are the sign and proof of the living virtue in it.
>
> Winston S. Churchill, quoted in Gilbert, 1991, pp. 214–215.

One of my graduate students, a physician, once asked in class "Why should we care about the health of these people [prisoners], considering what they've done?" It is a question that many people both inside and outside the prison system may legitimately ask. Such a question is sometimes a function of the emotion associated with a reaction to a particularly distressing crime eclipsing a rational consideration of the principles and evidence regarding health care in prison settings. This chapter addresses the question posed through examining medical, penological, religious, public health and human rights principles in prison health care.

Modern public health also contributes, often unwittingly, to the belief that illness is not only linked to, and consequent upon, poor behavior, but thus deserved. The connection between smoking and lung and other cancers and pulmonary disease, between poor diet and obesity and many cancers, between sexual behavior and HIV and STDs, and alcohol and drug consumption and accidents and violence are all well proven. It is a small step to go beyond health behaviors to "blaming the victim" (Ryan, 1976) for their subsequent illness. If Samuel Butler was writing his satirical criminological novel *Erewhon* today, one might expect his "straighteners" to be acting as triage at emergency departments, allocating patients from ambulances on the basis of their perceived responsibility for their illness. Indeed, there would probably be a close correspondence between blameworthiness and allocation to a purgatory department to await care the longest. Such views of blameworthiness, whether from a religious or a health perspective, appear to underlie the dismissal of decent health care in prisons as justified. The nexus between poor health and the prison population, based on widely demonstrated linkages between lower social class and poorer health, however, may on the contrary justify the application of a "correctional' model rather than a punitive model to health care in jails and prisons.

The "just world" phenomenon (Lerner and Simmons, 1966) describes the perception that when bad things happen to people, they must have deserved them, since the world is essentially just. Allied to this concept is the conception, frequently subliminal, but based on centuries of Judeo-Christian teaching, that poor health is at worst a punishment for sins, or at best a trial to be stoically borne. In the Bible, the book of Job illustrates the determination of Job's friends that he must have sinned to deserve his suffering (even though no such sin is apparent to them). Despite this, it transpires that this is a test for Job from God, not a punishment. Likewise, in the New Testament, Christ responds to the question as to who had sinned, the man born blind or his parents, to result in his having been born blind. The response, again similar to that toward Job, is that neither had sinned (but that he was born blind so that the works of God might be revealed in him: John 9:1–3). These passages theologically show illness not as "deserved," but quite the opposite. However, these popular responses to illness as being "deserved" also reveal a deep-seated common assumption that sickness is a punishment for sin. It is a small (and dangerous) step to take to see the health problems of prisoners as somehow "deserved." Indeed, it may validate the "just world" perception, since prisoners are obviously bad.

On giving good care to bad people

There is no penological benefit to providing poor or negligent health care to inmates.[1] Yet a common response to poor health care in prisons is that inmates don't "deserve" good health care. Such an approach largely emerges from a "just desserts" approach to punishment, where there is a lack of sympathy for restrictive environments in correctional facilities – essentially, the view that there needs to be a level of suffering inherent in a custodial sentence. Deprivation of liberty on its own is seen as being insufficient, and there additionally needs to be an environment of deprivation. Justice (as punishment) not only needs to be done, but needs to be seen to be done. Thus, reasonable conditions (of which health care is seen to be part and parcel) are perceived as being contrary to just desserts.

Correctional health

While we widely use the term "correctional" with regard to jail and prison settings, we still tend to see the "corrections" as primarily occurring as a result of the deprivation of liberty. Many correctional settings also seek to reform (or "correct") the antisocial or maladaptive behaviors that lead to the crime in the first place. It is increasingly recognized that such behaviors cannot be seen in isolation from deprived backgrounds or mental illness – in short, environmental and medical factors that share common roots with the same health deficits that are over-represented in prisoners. If correction can extend to mental health issues, given that courts make little if any distinction between mental and physical illness, then it should also extend to correcting health issues that, like future criminal behavior, will be a major cost to the community. With over half of inmates re-offending and returning to prison, small amounts of preventive health education may also have future savings in later incarcerations, at a direct saving to the criminal justice system. It does not take a very broad change in the conception of "correctional" programs to extend from mental to physical health, with emphasis on future costs to the community, whether directly through prison medical care, or indirectly through health care. The case can be made that we should not only care, but care more, for inmates' health.

A human right to health care?

Health care in prison has been asserted to be a "human right." "Human rights" has become a commonplace (perhaps over-used) term which asserts that there is a moral force which ensures that people are treated with respect due to their inherent dignity and worth as a human (Clapham, 2007). Traditionally, human rights were seen as protections against arbitrary power, but have more recently been conceptualized as universally valid principles and standards of behavior with which human beings are endowed by reason of their humanity (status as a human) (Clapham, 2007, p. 5).

Clapham, however, notes that when the concept of human rights is applied to criminals, the issue becomes contentious. Accusations are made that the "rights" of criminals are ranked higher than those of law-abiding citizens (p. 3) and that the rule of law is somehow subverted by emphasizing the rights of the criminal or the accused. Largely, he argues, such accusations turn out on inspection to be sensationalist or based on inaccurate information, since human rights are considered a special, narrow category of rights: "*extraordinarily* special, basic interests" which sets them apart from rights, even moral rights, generally (p. 5). They are based on the universally valid principles and standards of behavior that human beings, by reason of being human, have fundamental and inalienable rights (that is, rights that are inherent in being human and cannot be removed).

These rights, argues the English writer Thomas Paine (1791), are based on the "reality of distress." A similar conception was used by Paine's contemporary Jeremy Bentham for the prevention of cruelty to animals: "The question is not, Can they *reason*? nor Can they *talk*? but, Can they *suffer*?" (Bentham, 1789). Thus, as Clapham (2007, pp. 20–21) observes, the justification for the primacy of human rights is that certain acts offend the conscience of humanity – and specifically, offend against our sense of common humanity and shared suffering. It is not predicated on the crimes or sins of the individual human, but on their shared humanity with us. Part of that shared humanity is the possession of a human body and faculties – the ability to feel pain and suffer distress. It is this "embodiment" – possession of a human body – that suggests that appropriate care of the body of prisoners may be one avenue to their humanization. If prisoners, whatever their crimes, also have an inherent value as humans, then appropriate care for their health needs becomes a form of "re-humanization." Rehabilitation (literally, "making fit again") can refer to the body as well as other abilities or behaviors.

One of the major gaps in rehabilitation of prisoners is the absence of rehabilitation of the body. Inmates are at a major disadvantage with regard to their health and disease status due to the stratum of the community they come from, and the frequent lack of access to health services through barriers of availability, cost and location. Providing the possibility of health rehabilitation through provision of treatment for existing disorders, screening and vaccination, and particularly through preventive education, should be an integral part of any comprehensive prison health service. Such health rehabilitation would have two beneficial impacts on the community when the offender re-enters the free world. First, the burden of disease or potential disease in the community may be reduced. Second, the individual may become an agent of diffusion of health information within a sector of the community that is at disproportionate risk for health problems. Health rehabilitation may not fall within the narrow range of what is traditionally and currently considered "what works" in rehabilitation (such as absence of re-offending or stable employment), although it is closer to current goals of prison-based effective and sustainable drug and alcohol treatment. Why should the rehabilitated body not be considered as much one of the legitimate goals of correctional facilities as the rehabilitated life? Indeed, it may actively contribute to the "genuine humanization of all" (Romero, 1988, p. 55), including more global aspects of the lifestyle of the offender.

Humanity and prison health care

One encounters the argument that many inmates are, by reason of the nature of the crimes they have committed, unworthy or less worthy of being considered fully human. The attractions of denying the humanity of particular individuals, based on a demonstrated lack of humanity in their own behavior to others, are tempting, but lead in dangerous directions. There is an understandable tendency, on hearing of a particularly violent or dreadful crime, to declare the perpetrator to be inhuman or less than human (crucially, this categorization establishes them as dissimilar to self) – and thus, not a candidate for treatment as a human. Such labeling as sub-human and its logical tendency was the focus of the war crimes tribunals set up following World War II. It was a necessary step in the development of the Holocaust that Jewish people first be defined by the Nazis as sub-human (*untermenschen*) before murdering them (along with other ethnic groups defined by the Nazis as "inferior races," such as Gypsies, Slavs and other classes of people deemed by them to be undesirable). By defining them as not human or less than human, human considerations such as prohibitions on cruelty, murder and torture did not apply. This may appear an extreme argument in the context of prison health, but consider the trials of the Nazi doctors in 1946, which provide the link between the political definition of a person as unworthy of treatment as a human, and punitive or inhumane medical treatment. In the quote at the beginning of this chapter, the famous conservative British statesman Sir Winston Churchill, leader of Britain in World War II, stated over 100 years ago that "the treatment of crime and criminals is one of the most unfailing tests of the civilization of any country," and that "the treatment of crime and criminals mark and measure the stored-up strength of a nation, and are the sign and proof of the living virtue in it."

The Nuremberg doctors' trials

The concept of crimes against humanity was introduced in the trial of the Nazi leaders at Nuremberg following World War II. The second Nuremberg trial was of Nazi doctors (Lifton, 2000; Schmidt, 2006, 2007; Spitz, 2005). A number of Nazi doctors and medical assistants were hanged and many imprisoned following their trial and conviction in this and the simultaneous Dachau medical trial, for crimes against humanity in the course of the Third Reich. While it is correct to note that these trials focused largely on mass murder by medical and health personnel and experimentation on prisoners without consent (leading to the Nuremberg Code for medical experimentation on humans), some crucial issues relating to medicine and imprisonment arose.

Lifton (2000, p. 186) notes the "healing–killing reversal" that the Nazi doctors engaged in to medically legitimize acts of inhumanity, injustice and murder in the Third Reich. Here, there was a caricature of triage which provided "an aura of healing" when the medical personnel were acting as agents of the state rather than as agents of medicine. The use of medical forms and terms served to legitimize their healing–killing reversal. Clearly, nothing so extreme occurs in correctional institutions that have properly trained medical and nursing staff in the developed world. However, there may be an analogy in a "healing–punishing reversal" that some health staff may feel socially or occupationally pressured into. In contrast, Lifton (2000, p. 238) notes that many Jewish and Polish prisoner-doctors in the Nazi concentration camps, themselves in danger of death, managed to provide comfort to the sick – they "remained doctors ... in spite of everything," dispensing the few aspirin available, and giving words of comfort and hope. This maintenance of the determination to try to heal even under the most extreme conditions impressed upon the prisoner-doctors how much they could actually do despite the immense limitations of medicine, facilities and freedom (Lifton, 2000, p. 504). It is a pertinent lesson for resource-deprived health settings.

One of the most difficult judgments that health care personnel have to make does not occur under the extreme conditions described by Lifton (2000) and Spitz (2005) in the Third Reich, but the principles derived from the Nuremberg doctors' trials are helpful. Who are the health staff working for – the justice system or the patient? Where does their allegiance lie? This argument was raised at the doctors' trials and the judgment and subsequent sentences made it clear that the Hippocratic Oath was not trumped by orders or perceived duties. The Hippocratic Oath (Spitz, 2005, pp. ix–x) refers to keeping the sick from harm *and injustice*, and lest it be thought that the reference to injustice is not central, Hippocrates further reiterates that the physician comes for the benefit of the sick, remaining *free of all intentional injustice* (my italics). The potential for health care to merge into injustice was as much a reality in Greek medicine as it is in medicine – particularly correctional medicine – today. As health personnel in correctional facilities, we have an ethical obligation, stemming from the Hippocratic Oath, to do no harm, to help the sick *and* to avoid injustice in their health care. Nowhere in the Hippocratic Oath or equivalent formulations of ethics is there any reference to whether the patient *deserves* care. It is easy to provide extreme cases to make a point – juxtaposing Winston Churchill and the Third Reich provides clarity to the conflict that highlighted those principles and the ideologies behind those principles. Yet the difficulties that face us in prison medicine are usually much more subtle.

Limitations of rights through legal process

Human and political rights may be limited through legal due process. Imprisonment removes liberty, and in some cases freedom of expression, of assembly, association and property. In some states, the criminal may not have the right to vote not only during their imprisonment, but also after release. In extreme cases, the law may provide for deprivation of life (execution). Why, then, should health care for inmates not also be considered limited by imprisonment?

First, punishment must have a legitimate aim in the interference with rights. It is hard to see condemnation to poor health or lack of treatment as having a legitimate legal aim given that punishments of the body and torture are widely considered in most countries as unacceptable penal methods. Second, the interference with rights should be prescribed by a clear and comprehensible law. It is rare that secular penal systems prescribe any form of corporal punishment, mutilation or torture in the twenty-first century, although it may still occur in some forms of religion-based law. Third, the interference with the right (in our case, denial of health care) should be proportionate to the identified legitimate aim, and necessary in a democratic society (Clapham, 2007), assuming that such proportionality can be measured. For this last point to be met, one would expect that the denial of health care would be proportionate to the crime rather than a random event that would produce a punishment based on the chance occurrence or not of illness in the prisoner, and the length and severity of that illness.

Duty of health care

The law establishes unequivocally in both the United States and the UK that there is a duty of health care for inmates. However, this duty of care is limited. In the UK it is equivalent to standard NHS service (and since prison medical services have now been taken over by the NHS, it should be indistinguishable from local NHS services). In the United States it is limited to immediate care for conditions that cannot be put off without undue pain or residual injury to the inmate – and not elective care. Given that 95 percent of US inmates lack health insurance, there are often concerns that inmates should not be seen to be getting better health care than they would receive in the free world – or in some way "benefiting" from being in prison. Thus, care of inmates is limited to obvious, symptomatic conditions, although in jails it is usual to screen new entrants for infectious diseases of public health importance, such as tuberculosis, syphilis and STDs such as Chlamydia and gonorrhea, which are notifiable and easily treatable. Other diseases that have high prevalence in prisons and are vaccinatable against such as Hepatitis B may also be screened for. Depending on the jurisdiction, and on often limited prison health care budgets, secondary prevention – screening for early detection of disease – may not be actively pursued, since the detection of a condition will bring with it an obligation to treat.

For preventive health care and health education there is no established legal duty of care. Nevertheless, many jurisdictions have comprehensive prevention programs, ranging from parenting classes to HIV prevention programs (e.g., Ross *et al.*, 2006). However, I would argue that from the third purpose of imprisonment – community protection – there is a clear duty of care for health education and health promotion. Classically, community protection is seen as the removal of people who endanger others in the community specifically, or generally in terms of their propensity to commit crime. However, beyond the specifics of individuals and criminal behaviors, one can see a more general obligation to protect the community from a general and public health class of harm that could be addressed at relatively low cost and with potentially high impact. Health education (which should be a voluntary activity) may be one of those health services where there is a duty of general care to protect the community against known higher risks for preventable health conditions. At its most specific, this entails *risk reduction* education.

A duty of risk reduction education?

The high prevalence of HIV and Hepatitis B in prison inmates reflects both sexual and drug-related risk behaviors, and we have a duty of care to the public to prevent both those inmates already infected from infecting others on release, and those who are uninfected from becoming infected, given their high level of risk behaviors. Thus, risk reduction education for preventing HIV and Hepatitis B and C transmission through injecting drug use (need for new needles and syringes, or cleaning by bleach of used needles and syringes if new ones are not available) is a clear community protection for a class of individuals at high risk. Indeed, it is a community protection largely tied to the drug-related offences which frequently (directly or indirectly) lead to their imprisonment. It should be made available along with more traditional, individually directed risk reduction interventions for individual prisoners, such as drug treatments, which are essentially reducing risk through *demand reduction*. Second, given high sexual risk behaviors leading to HIV and other STD infection, risk reduction education involving situationally focused risk awareness and condom education and promotion constitutes community protection from a highly foreseeable set of risks. While it might be argued from a legal standpoint that it is not usually possible to tie particular individuals to health risks when released (except in a statistical sense), it is possible to tie inmates to increased public health risks. Such a calculation of risks is akin to that which is made on the potential of an individual to re-offend, in making decisions on their release. If a community had a group of people – prisoners or in the free world – at significantly increased risk of disease, then public health programs would be directed at those groups wherever possible. Thus, I argue that there is a specific duty of care for health risk reduction education to inmates for the protection of the community, and a more general one to make available the same types of risk reduction health education programs to inmates as are available to the general community. In the first case, we have a specific knowledge of the need for risk reduction, frequently based upon the offences for which the inmate has been imprisoned (drug use, offences associated with obtaining drug money) or their infection with HIV or Hepatitis B or C. In the more general second case, we have a population at high statistical risk of disease, who should be able to benefit from public health programs to the same extent as the rest of the community.

Legitimacy: beyond fairness and decency

There are good reasons to treat prisoners with fairness. Not only are fairness and decency rated as one of the most important dimensions of prison climate by both correctional staff *and* prisoners (Liebling and Arnold, 2004), but prison staff are important role models to prisoners for appropriate behavior. Punitive treatment of prisoners fails to take into account that, first, about half of prisoners are in prison for non-violent offenses, and second, that about half will not re-offend. What sort of appropriate behavior is modeled for prisoners who will return to society? That is up to prison staff. If prisoners cannot distinguish between the unstable and violent behavior of other prisoners and the behavior of some prison staff, they may perceive that such behavior is the norm. Liebling and Arnold (2004, p. 471) make the point that fairness and decency *legitimize* incarceration. Legitimacy provides the moral credibility of imprisonment to the inmate and to prison staff. Whatever removes that legitimacy degrades prison authority to that of abuse of power by just another gang.

Haney (2005) comments on his shock on seeing a billboard at a church outside a prison in the United States which read "Compassion in the face of evil is no virtue." Not only is such a statement offensive to most faiths, but it confuses *bad* and *evil*. Very few people in prison could be described as totally evil: the vast majority will have redeeming features which merit an attempt to cultivate or support the positive in them. This benefits both the prison environment (including staff and prisoner safety), *and* the community upon re-entry. Treating prisoners as human can, at a minimum, model and reinforce its appropriateness for their own human interactions (Maruna, 2001). What is "correctional" about modeling behaviors that Haney refers to as "uncaring, or brutalizing" (2005, p. 68)? Compassion may not be crucial to fairness and decency, but fairness and decency are crucial to legitimacy, whether it is legitimacy of the authority of prison custodial staff or of health care professionals.

Good health care can *increase* legitimacy, through providing a model of care for persons and for the powerless. It can also give legitimacy *to health care*, in providing preventive and timely care that is not sought at the point of serious disease or pain, and is given in a professional and caring manner.

The Declaration of Moscow

The Declaration of Moscow of October 24, 2003, is a World Health Organization declaration (WHO, 2003) on prison health as a part of public health. Its guiding principles include the United Nations (UN) Basic Principles for the Treatment of Prisoners, and the UN Principles of Medical Ethics Relevant to the Role of Health Personnel, in the Protection of Prisoners and Detainees. Its guiding principles further recognize that the act of depriving a person of liberty "always entails a duty of care which calls for effective methods of prevention, screening and treatment." That is, we have a *special* duty of care to inmates, because by depriving them of their liberty, we also deprive them of the freedom to engage in health care on their own behalf should they choose to access it. And since health care cannot be tied to the pains of imprisonment (indeed, denial of health care to an inmate may constitute cruel and unusual punishment), we have a duty of care to ensure that "all necessary health care for those deprived of their liberty" (p. 3) is available to inmates since we have deprived them of access to it. Health care is specifically *not* one of the recognized deprivations of liberty entailed in imprisonment or detention.

The Declaration of Moscow identifies specific problems that lead to absent or substandard health care in prisons. Their remediation includes joint training of prison health and prison security personnel, continuity of treatment between prison and the free world, treatment that is free, and making harm reduction the guiding principle of policy. Consistently, the *Declaration* also recognizes that appropriate protection for prison staff from health hazards is equally an obligation of governments. Prisoner education and disease prevention is recognized as an urgent need. Psychiatric and psychological treatments are emphasized as being of central importance, along with physical health issues, and the particular problem of infectious diseases spreading in confined spaces is raised. Finally, the requirement to meet minimum environmental standards for light, space, air, water and nutrition in prisons is noted.

While the Declaration of Moscow is phrased as a series of recommendations, it is firmly situated in the framework of UN covenants on rights, principles and ethics. And while the recommendations are phrased in terms of public health imperatives, it is significant that the justifications for these are primarily based on human rights. Having deprived prisoners of the opportunity to obtain health care in the free world, whatever its standard, we have taken upon ourselves a duty of care (that is, the responsibility to provide) for the health of those inmates as long as they are in our custody. This is not optional, nor is it based on what sort of health care is the norm in the free world. Indeed, the Declaration makes the point that from a purely health-based perspective, inmates disproportionately include the most vulnerable to disease and those with the poorest health, and thus those for whom there should be a preferential option for health care.

We can see, therefore, that giving good care to bad people has very little to do with the actual or alleged moral standing or criminal behavior of the inmate or detainee. It has nothing to do with punishment, even if we had the right to impose our own punishments in addition to those of the courts. What it has to do with is issues of humanity – the status of the inmate as human, and equally with our response to them as reflecting on our *own* humanity. Finally, there is a rehabilitative health imperative, for the good of both the wider community and of prison staff, to prevent and contain disease and poor health – regardless of our views about the individual carrier of that disease. Being human does not come with degrees of humanity or with special conditions, or depend on how much we like someone, but is an absolute. We give good care to bad people because we are professional, and because we, and they, are human. To the extent that we give bad care, the humanity that we degrade is also ours, not only theirs.

6 Pedagogy for prisoners

An approach to peer health education for inmates[1]

"The body as the major target of penal repression has disappeared," according to Foucault (1977, p. 8). While punishment has become a hidden process, with prison a non-corporal penalty, the emphasis is on correction, reclamation and "cure" of the prisoner (Foucault, 1977, p. 10). Nevertheless, Foucault also notes the hold on the body remains. Additional elements of punishment – rationing of food, sexual deprivation, corporal punishment and solitary confinement – to name some of these elements, have what he calls "unintentional but inevitable" (p. 16) consequences for the body. While Foucault is correct in noting that the body is no longer the direct target of the penal system, the change in punishment–body relations is by no means absolute. Turner (1996) has noted that the institutionalization of the body, with increasing control of daily life, defines a corporeal existence through the bodily functions of "eating, washing, grooming, dressing and sleeping" (p. 37) (all of which are controlled in prisons). Inmates are limited in the ability to express their personal needs through constructing their bodies, since prison regimes limit consumption, ownership, pleasure and desire, movement, diet and conditions of excretion. Regulation of the body, at least for adults, is often at its most extreme in prisons. Individual expression using the body may be limited to an exercised body and tattoos: thus, the body and its functions are the object of control, though not usually of formal punishment.

While the body itself is not the primary target of the penal system, it could be argued that the body of the prisoner is frequently still a *devalued* body, with consequences for health – both morbidity and, in extreme cases, mortality. While these are unintentional, a secondary result of imprisonment, they may impact the health of the prisoner through a number of mechanisms. These may include residual informal violence in prisoners, from fellow prisoners or from staff (the latter usually idiosyncratic although its encouragement or discouragement may vary considerably from system to system and unit to unit); harms from the environment, particularly in facilities with old construction, overcrowding and poor ventilation and sanitary systems; self-harm on the part of inmates, such as injecting drugs, tattooing, sexual behavior and use of cell-brewed liquor; and organizational harm as a function of poor prison social and moral climates which view the devalued inmate body as unworthy of appropriate health care (Sim, 1990). Nevertheless, it would be a mistake to blame the health issues of inmates in the correctional system solely on the system itself: the inmate typically comes from an underclass with poor health and access to health care. There is thus a tension between the *importation* of poor health and its *production* (or *reduction*) in any penal system. Relevant here is the impact of imprisonment itself on the inmate body. Inmates may engage in potentially or actually health-debilitating behaviors (such as drug use and other risk behaviors) to self-medicate or to dull the pains of imprisonment, or because such risky behaviors are an integral part of the inmate prison culture. Whether an inmate leaves in better or worse health is a function of a balance of multiple levels of factors ranging from the population through the system and individual level. However, it would be a mistake to assume that because the spectacle of the body *as object of* punishment has disappeared, the body *as subject to* the impact of imprisonment has also disappeared. The body as object of rehabilitation is beginning to emerge, and a health education and literacy approach to health rehabilitation is the subject of this chapter.

This chapter reviews data on the public health status of prisoners both inside and outside correctional environments, and the significance of the prison in providing public health services that benefit both the prisoner and the community to which they return. I describe the importance of prison preventive health education using Freire's (1972) critical pedagogy model, and its potential secondary consequences for inmate health literacy and self-efficacy. Finally, I discuss the importance of prison health education as part of a wider "healthy prisons" approach to provision of health literacy for the under-served.

Prisoners largely represent the lowest socioeconomic strata of society, and the operation of Hart's (1971) "inverse care law": that those with most need of medical treatment have the poorest access to it. However, in many correctional systems which exist in places with no or minimal health care available without cost, it can be argued that the inmate enjoys *better* health care in prison than their peers in the "free world." There is thus a contrast between a place such as Britain, where there is basic health care available to all and the goal is to bring prison health care up to NHS standards (HMPS/ NHS, 1999), and the United States, where over 90 percent of inmates are medically uninsured (Conklin *et al.*, 1998) and may paradoxically receive *better* care in a correctional setting (although the services may still be substandard) than in the free world. I call this paradox of prison health care in relation to its free world health care setting the "perverse care law." In the United States such enhanced care in prisons may result from legal challenges to the standard of correctional health care, as in the case of *Ruiz* v. *Estelle* (1980) in Texas.

By conventional measures of formal employment, perhaps only one-third of the prison population is formally employed at time of arrest, and in terms of education and literacy, prisoners have low literacy rates. Indeed, prisoners frequently come from an underclass of the socially excluded, the unemployed and the working poor, who have been in this situation for several generations. Young (2002) argues that the unemployed are denied a basic economic substratum concomitant with the expectations of what "citizenship" implies; the working poor are denied it by the unfair hours worked and remuneration. Thus, prisoners are far more likely to be situated as a "functional underclass" at the lowest socioeconomic stratum of society. In terms of all forms of literacy (prose, documentary and quantitative literacy), US prisoners of both genders, all race/ethnicities and all age groups score significantly lower than those in households (Greenberg *et al.*, 2007), although the levels of literacy in prisoners rose between 1992 and 2003. They are also very significantly disadvantaged in health status.

Social status and health

There is a substantial body of research that establishes that people in the lowest strata of society have significantly lower health, on a number of indices, than those at higher socioeconomic and social-class levels (Wilkinson, 1996): indeed, the relationship is essentially linear by class (Townsend *et al.*, 1988). In a large cohort of Scottish men, Hart *et al.* (1998) established that this relationship between lower social-class level and mortality, measured at childhood, labor market entry and screening, remained similar at each stage, with the higher social classes having the lowest risk, especially for all causes of death and cardiovascular disease, suggesting that the risk–social class relationship is maintained throughout the life course. This risk–social class relationship was shown to be stable across ten western and Scandinavian countries (Kunst *et al.*, 2005), with increases in inequalities for women, and for all countries except for the Scandinavian ones. It seems that these Nordic countries' welfare states are able to buffer many of the adverse effects of economic disadvantage on the health of disadvantaged groups. Kunst *et al.* note that health inequalities are deeply rooted in the social stratification systems of modern societies. Further, the social class gap for preventive health behaviors, a major precursor to morbidity and mortality, also appears to be widening: Alvarez-Dardet *et al.* (2001) studied lifestyle choices in the Spanish national health surveys over a decade and found that for smoking, alcohol consumption, physical exercise and obesity, the disadvantaged population worsened on all these indices, while the more affluent groups exhibited a net gain on all these indices. Thus, health risk behaviors in the most disadvantaged classes appear to be worsening, which will almost certainly lead to an exacerbation of the social class divide in morbidity and mortality. Correctional facilities may thus serve as important institutions for health delivery and health promotion to populations most at risk and most in need.

Healthy prisons and prison health education

The concept of "healthy prisons" which was originally launched by the World Health Organization (Smith, 2000) was introduced in the UK by Lord Ramsbotham as Chief Inspector of Prisons (HMIP, 1996; Ramsbotham, 2003). The tension in the concept of "healthy prisons" has been analyzed by Smith (2000), who notes that while there is general agreement that prisons should be sites for the promotion of health, it could be described as part of "surveillance medicine," with activities directed toward the management of the population's health. She argues that "the responsibility for both the *cause* and the *cure* of health problems becomes firmly located in the individual, deflecting attention away from the wider social structure which both *creates* some behaviors and *inhibits* the development and maintenance of others" (p. 343; italics in original). Thus, for many prisoners, health promotion directives may be meaningless or may be seen as a health agenda imposed by the authorities. There is also, as Smith recognizes, a tension between attempting to promote personal empowerment in an environment in which very little individual choice and responsibility can be permitted by prison staff, including prison health care workers.

Prison education has traditionally, suggests Collins (1988), been based on making available to inmates educational and training opportunities. Collins notes three models: the medical model, which sees education and training as reparative of criminality and which will reduce recidivism; the "opportunities" model to keep inmates busy and provide vocational skills; and the cognitive deficiency model. This latter model "assumes that shortcomings in the inmates' way of knowing and acting are associated with a perpetration of inappropriate actions that cause harm and injury to others" (Collins, 1988, p. 105). Collins characterizes all these approaches, including self-directed learning, as serving to shape and normalize the actions of inmates through adult education. Collins argues that self-directed learning is simply a panoptic (surveillance and control-based) method applied to the shaping of behavior, but also suggests that Freire's (1972) pedagogic model may provide one option to panoptic models of prison education.

In this chapter I propose an approach to prison health education that is minimally related to direct reduction in recidivism, occupying inmates' time or vocational skills training, but addresses the health disparities associated with the disadvantaged in general and prisoners in particular. It is emancipatory from a personal health and community health perspective, and situates the participant as a peer educator both inside and outside of the correctional environment. Smith (2000) has noted that there is a contradiction between the levels of control and minimalization of personal responsibility in prisons, and promoting personal empowerment in health. This tension, however, may be a facilitator of health promoting education in prisons, because health promotion, provided its content is generated by the participants and not imposed by the authorities, may be one of the few occasions open to inmates for the legitimate exercise of personal choice, development of skills as peer educators and empowerment. Indeed, health enfranchisement may be one of the few avenues open for prisoners to build a sense of achievement and self-worth in a system which frequently treats them as worthless or devalues their worth. One appropriate model for prison health education may be Freire's pedagogic model.

Pedagogy for prisoners

Paulo Freire's (1972) concept of education as humanizing (emancipating) involves people becoming autonomous and responsible, rather than following an imposed prescription of behavior. He refers to traditional pedagogy as the "pedagogy of the oppressed" and as being characterized by "banking education." Freire's approach to humanizing education is centered around his rejection of such "banking education," in which the teacher makes a "deposit" of knowledge which the student is expected to "withdraw" and repeat in an examination. In "banking education" the teacher presents a reality that is static and compartmentalized, filling the students with contents detached from their reality and without significance to them. Such an approach, Freire argues, usually bears no relationship to the student's immediate life situation and needs, or indeed relevance to this situation: indeed, "banking education" may kill curiosity, creativity and the investigative spirit in students.

In contrast, "problematizing education" is a dialogue between the educator and the student, where both learn together as a collective project. Here, there is an active relationship between knowledge and the knower, in contrast to the passive reception of often irrelevant information in the "banking" approach (Freire, 1972). Freire suggests that abstract concepts are also frequently irrelevant to the concrete situation and social structure that learners face, partly because they do not use the language of the student, partly because they are not discussing the learner's own situation, environment and immediate needs – what he calls "insertion in the social context" (Gadotti, 1994, p. 9). Freire (1972, p. 48) indicates that the marginalized are not living "outside" society, but have always been members of it. Transforming education so that it is relevant to the marginalized and allows them to become "beings for themselves" (humanized) is one of the central goals of problematizing education. Prisoners represent some of the most marginalized individuals in western society, and problematizing education appears a highly relevant approach to education in correctional settings. Its success with other disadvantaged communities in South America and Africa has been widely demonstrated (Taylor, 1993; Gadotti, 1994).

Gadotti notes that for the learner, the production of new knowledge is not as important as the *discovery* of that knowledge. In traditional "banking" education, the teacher is the specialist in transferring knowledge. However, in Freire's approach, the discovery changes the locus of control from the teacher to the student. Central to his pedagogy, Freire argues, is the choice of themes and topics by the learners. The educator can add themes as fundamental elements in this choice which could clarify or expand the theme proposed by the people's group. Teaching, according to Freire, is a partnership between teacher and student in which both may be learners, and not an authoritarian system in which content is prescribed and students filled with information, and where they are not respected as contributing participants. However, as Gadotti (1994, p. 57) notes, using the format of a dialogue does not mean that the educator is non-directive, but just non-manipulative – directing without ordering.

Prior to any educative exercise, the teacher needs to carry out formative work to understand the language and idiom, world view, and the problems lived by the group, in order to generate the themes and concepts necessary to have effective education. This is especially important not only for basic literacy but also for health literacy, where the conception of health and illness and their causative factors is critical to building an understanding of the body and control of health. Crucial here is the concept of *conscientização*, conscientization: "developing consciousness, but consciousness that is understood to have the power to transform reality" (Taylor 1993, p. 52). For Freire, this means developing not only an understanding of what, for example in health literacy, causes illness or maintains health, but understanding what needs to be changed and what is within one's power to change.

Teachers themselves must also be quite familiar with the area to be covered. Freire stressed the need for the one who is "teaching" to know the material in depth – so as not to rob the student of the historical, political and philosophical background in which a well-thought-out theory or argument is based. This involves knowing in depth not only the particular point of view to which the teacher subscribes, but also the opposing points of view. This implies a thorough reading and understanding of the positions of those who are in opposition, so as to have a clear conception of one's arguments, their failings and contradictions, and through a dialectic approach being able to create a new synthesis that will possibly change and improve the original position (Ferreira-Pinto, personal communication).

While it is argued that Freire's approach is not a method (Freire and Macedo, 1993), Gadotti (1994) nevertheless notes that this approach has three stages. First, in the *investigation* stage, there is a qualitative investigation of the universe of the students' vocabulary and current concepts about the universe of the problem, and their experiences in the area. As an example, stories about experiences in health can illustrate students' concept of control of health, and what can lead to positive or negative outcomes, and most important, why. The words, concepts, and problems arising from experiences become the material for the next stage, *thematization*.

In *thematization* the themes arising from the previous stage are expanded. For example, in health education and health promotion, new generative themes and concepts may emerge, such as immunization, diet, exercise, disease transmission, organ function and treatment, to be dealt with as subjects for investigation from the perspective of the student and of control of their health and its maintenance, or control over treatment options.

In the third stage, *problematization*, these themes are moved from the abstract to the concrete. Here, *conscientization*, critical consciousness, develops: "The oppressive reality is experienced as a process that can be overcome" (Gadotti, 1994, p. 23). In the health field, specific examples of health problems that were generated from the thematization and from a list of topics of concern to the students that arose in the first two stages can be addressed with emphasis on how a degree of control over health – through prevention, screening and treatment – can be achieved. Gadotti (1994, p. 23) calls this a transformative praxis: a collectively organized act of education with emphasis on the subject (that is, the student). The problems become not only problems with the patient as a passive object, but issues where the student can understand the factors that lead to control of the health problems and often have a degree of control over them. This is best illustrated by a concrete example in a prison system.

As an initial stage, what I have called *identification*, it is important to meet with participants to elicit information as to what health issues are important to them. An example of this appears in Table 6.1. After a session on HIV prevention with inmates in the Ciudad Juárez prison in Chihuahua, México, we asked inmates: If they had an opportunity to study and understand health problems that concern them, what those issues might be.[2] Inmates were vocal and enthusiastic in their descriptions of health issues they wanted to know about, and generated the topics listed in the Table in less than five minutes.

Table 6.1 Identification of health areas of concern generated by inmates in Ciudad Juárez prison

---

Hepatitis B, Hepatitis C
Human papilloma virus infection (genital warts, cervical cancer)
Tuberculosis
Diabetes
Myocardial infarction, hypertension
Arthritis
Sports injuries (knees, hands, feet)
Skin diseases
Depression, suicidal ideation
Stress-related diseases (colitis, gastrointestinal symptoms)
Epilepsy, convulsions
Aging and geriatric health
First aid and CPR

Note:
$n = 25$ men, 3 women, inmate peer educators in HIV prevention class.

Let us assume that blood pressure is one of the topics that came up, either directly or in terms of problems that are associated with high blood pressure (hypertension) or its associated medications. Then, in the *investigation* stage, it is important to elicit "folk constructions" – what students understand by blood pressure problems and what they understand its health and quality of life impacts to be. Often, popular understanding contains misconceptions or myths. Then we need to elicit what is understood about the cardiovascular system and how it works, again with emphasis on what is accurate and what is inaccurate. What popular analogies are used to understand the cardiovascular system? Sometimes the analogy of a pump is used. This might be expanded to explain the problems associated with high blood pressure – for example, high pressure and rubber hoses that are weak or worn out (or a pump with limited power and high resistance). This is *thematization*.

Next, *problematization* occurs – what health issues arise from problems with blood pressure, and from its associated medications? At this point, *conscientization* will be occurring as we discuss the modifiable factors that are associated with high blood pressure – diet, salt intake, weight, smoking, exercise, stress and medication adherence, among others. Many of these are to a greater or lesser degree under the control of the student. In the prison context, however, there may be additional lack of control, such as limitations on food available, or exercise opportunities. What conscientization does, however, is create an awareness of the possibility of exercising some individual control over the body and health, and this can be followed up by discussing individual plans for reducing risk, both in prison and out in the "free world." What is occurring is a process of both health literacy and of taking what control over the health issue is possible under the circumstances. In the health context, Freire has noted (Gadotti, 1994, p. 26) that abstractions are to be avoided as illnesses are presented: he specifies that we should always focus on the concrete reality that is to be transformed.

The mechanism through which such education takes place, according to Freire, is dialogue. Dialogue is not just a tactic to achieve results, but a central category of education – it is human nature to discover and share through dialogue, and learning is a social process in which dialogue is the cement (Gadotti, 1994, p. 29). Through this dialogue, critical consciousness, awareness of the possibility of change – which leads to what we have come to refer to as self-efficacy (Bandura, 1986) – is the key concept. Bandura has emphasized that there can only be a sense of self-efficacy where the behavior is under the control of the individual. In a prison context, there are many conditions and behaviors that are not under the control of the individual, whether environmental or personal. Nevertheless, there are also almost always possibilities for exercising control over health conditions, however minimal, in correctional settings, and to a greater extent on release.

While critical consciousness is conceptualized as a liberation from domination, in health education it largely consists of a move from being dominated by a medical model (in which the health provider instructs the patient, or in some cases does not even do this, but simply orders a course of treatment), to understanding the problem and choosing to deal with it. Part of this involves a move away from waiting until there is an illness and passively following the prescribed treatment (what in public health is referred to as tertiary prevention), to taking control of the body as much as possible, in a preventive or ameliorative approach (referred to as primary or secondary prevention). In prison health, in an environment where issues of control are central to the operation of the correctional environment, there are likely to be more limits on healthy behavior than in the free world. However, in an environment where inmates are subject to close scrutiny and organization, health may be one of the few avenues open to them to maintain personal control. It may thus achieve a greater significance in prison. Finally, it is always important to discuss health in the context not only of prison but of the free world. Ninety-five percent of prisoners will be released from prison at some point in time, and they need to consider healthy lifestyles in the free world as well as in prison. Further, prisoners, through visits with family and friends, also act as educators and models for significant numbers of people outside of the correctional environment: Ross *et al.* (2006) noted that over the course of a year, a group of HIV peer educators in the Texas prison system could potentially have educational contacts with over 80,000 individuals. Such contacts usually take the form of dialogues.

Dialogues with body and place

Freire has described the importance of a dialogue in his approach to education, but in the context of health education, he has also described it as a dialogue between the individual and their body (João Ferreira-Pinto, personal communication). Illness or pain is the body telling the individual that they have exceeded the limits of the system – Freire used the example of the symptoms of gout, resulting from excessive uric acid buildup in the joints, as his body telling him that he needed to restrict parts of his diet and to drink only one glass of red wine each week. Thus, when we talk of dialogue as a critical part of education, that dialogue is not just with educators and the rest of the class, but also an internal conversation with the body, in which the body can protest.

A second form of dialogue that Freire also emphasized as "problematizing" was interrogation of the environment. We can ask participants to look around and describe what they see that is of relevance to the topic broadly under discussion. For example, in a health context, we can ask the students to describe the environment that is seen and experienced and how it may have implications for health. Such an environment could include factors that might lead to stress, injury, depression, poor diet, lack of hygiene, or conversely factors that might lead to positive outcomes such as social interaction, opportunities for exercise, mental occupation and so on. The fact that such a vision in a correctional environment may be limited in no way invalidates the importance of interrogating the environment to form a critical consciousness of things that might be modified to impact health and provide some sense of personal control over one's body and health (whether short term or longer term). We need to recognize the limits, however, of history and social structures both inside and outside the prison, on health-related behaviors.

Health behaviors and history, culture and organizational context

Health education for inmates must take into account at least two of the barriers that Martín-Baró (1994) noted may occur in the application of psychological theories that were developed in wealthy and middle-class communities, to those from disadvantaged backgrounds. "Ahistoricism" presents the individual as bereft of history, community and society. Developing healthy behaviors in inmates must take account of their differing subjective and objective experiences, and recognize that what is valued as healthy or unhealthy is grounded in historical factors, both individual and collective. These may range from familial, community and spiritual folk remedies, as practiced by *curanderos* (traditional folk healers or shamans in Latin America), or adapting the role of the *curandero* to the correctional environment – for example, as a peer health leader. Unhealthy behaviors (for example, dietary habits, douching) may be firmly anchored in historical conditions that need to be recognized as having been adaptive, responding intuitively to a perceived health threat, or culturally or historically significant. Folk medicine may act as either a barrier or facilitator in health behavior change, but in either case needs to be treated as an integral part of the history and culture of health and disease in the investigation stage.

Second, Martín-Baró notes, problems are embedded in a matrix of social structures. Health behaviors, especially health-seeking behaviors and health risk behaviors require an understanding of the social and administrative structures (and barriers) and specifically the situations that frequently prevent accessing preventive and screening services (Ross and Ferreira-Pinto, 2000). When we teach about health in a correctional environment, much of that teaching will need to be about how to access health services in the free world – where to go, what to ask, how to deal with getting health service entitlement cards, registering with a health service, or what the language of health care is. Understanding how to be healthy involves equal parts of understanding the body and understanding the established administrative services and their location. There is little sense in moving toward early intervention and prevention if screening and immunization are unattainable. Thus, sessions that focus on *approaching* and *negotiating* health within existing health structures will be crucial. As an example, understanding how to get a county health card, when to access a community health clinic versus an emergency room, what immunizations are provided free and what they will (and won't) do, are as crucial to healthy living as understanding the effect of obesity on the heart. From Freire's and Martín-Baró's perspectives, then, eliciting issues about health access where health structures are obstructive or opaque are as crucial to achieving and maintaining health as eliciting health concerns where bodies are sick or dysfunctional. Approaching and negotiating health services can often be most effectively illustrated by dramatization.

Dramatization

Ross and Ferreira-Pinto (2000) argue that threats to health occur in settings and situations, rather than as decontextualized behaviors. The concept of the risk *situation* was recognized by Ross and Kelly (2000) as being important to address in reducing HIV risk – for example, drug users injecting without access to uncontaminated needles and syringes, alcohol or drugs associated with sex leading to lack of condom use, and issues of emotion, power or poverty leading to lack of protection. Thus, it is important to look at health risks being embedded in social and physical situations that may seriously compromise the degrees of freedom of the actor in that situation. As Goffman (1956) has noted with regard to many social behaviors, most behaviors become scripted. Including the development of unhealthy scripts and alternative (more healthy) scripts in any health program is essential for the actors to understand that health behaviors are staged in social situations and played out in social settings – and how to understand the usually invisible forces that maintain unhealthy behaviors and limit healthy options.

For correctional populations, I add an additional stage to Freire's model of pedagogy: *dramatization*. Freire (1972) has commented that "dramatization acts as a codification, as a problem-posing situation to be discussed" (p. 122). Since, as he argues, human activity consists of action and reflection, dramatization may form a "pre-praxis" where the lessons learned may be rehearsed to gain fluency and confidence in a safe environment. Health-seeking behaviors usually occur in a social setting, and frequently one with a significant imbalance of power. Setting up a situation in which scripts (in the sense that Goffman [1956] talks of the social actor's roles that are established and played) are developed, acted out and modified gives inmates an opportunity to model and familiarize themselves with interactions with health providers. These are *their* scripts, generated from personal experience, and the educator will work with them to produce and modify them. It is useful to integrate into scripts the concepts of both sides of the health equation: rights and responsibilities, services and behavior.

Articulating rights and responsibilities

The question of rights and responsibilities regarding health services for prisoners has been a matter of considerable debate. Generally, legal cases which address prison health issues (e.g., *Ruiz* v. *Estelle*, 1980, 503 F.Supp. 1295) hold that the state has a responsibility to provide health care that is of a standard equivalent to care provided outside the correctional system. While such a debate will largely depend on the jurisdiction and the level of health care available in the surrounding community, issues of health rights and health responsibilities are an important topic for consideration in health education in correctional institutions. "Rights" are usually balanced by associated "responsibilities" with regard to health. Seeing health care as a "right" may, paradoxically, reduce the perception of a personal "responsibility" for one's own health as important to them and those who depend on them. Further, responsibilities may also be active in the absence of clearly recognized rights. One of the areas that is a fruitful topic for consideration relates to the inmate's responsibility for their own health, in parallel with the responsibility of the prison system to provide health care. The responsibilities debate is important because it serves to link individual behaviors with health outcomes – for example, smoking, exercise, obesity, to name but a few. The usual outcome of this debate is to underscore the level of personal responsibility – often in an environment where the state assumes control of most aspects of daily life – for some personal issues such as health. While for major and catastrophic illness the state should and does take responsibility for care, balancing health rights and responsibilities can challenge a sense of fatalism and lack of control regarding health matters, and re-focus on the possibility of taking control of at least some areas of the body. Prisoner health literacy and, by extension, health education can thus become an integral part of public health interventions for the marginalized.

Public health as part of a continuum of care

From this, it is logical to look at public health interventions to reduce risk, as contrasted with tertiary care (treatment). Public health classically considers health as falling into three areas: primary care, avoiding a health condition before it occurs; secondary care, screening to detect early disease while it is still treatable and possibly before it reaches a severe stage; and tertiary care, treatment for illness when it has already become serious enough to seek medical attention. For an HIV-related example, primary prevention might involve promoting condoms to prevent HIV infection; secondary prevention might involve screening to detect HIV infection to treat it early; and tertiary prevention might involve treating full AIDS when it has debilitated the body and allowed opportunistic infections to disable the individual. Obviously, the further one goes from primary toward secondary prevention, and onto tertiary treatment, the more difficult and costly the condition is to treat, and the more the individual suffers from ill-health.

For many people, it is not until an illness becomes salient or unmanageable that care is sought. One of the central principles of health education for prisoners is that there are significant points of intervention and control *before* seeking medical treatment, and many of these are located in the domain of the individual, not the physician or nurse. For every health issue raised by the inmate, there should be a specific contemplation of the three public health stages: primary – "prevent"; secondary – "catch early"; tertiary – "treat late." It is an understanding of the *stages* of health and illness and their *progression*, as well as the *mechanisms*, which will provide a critical consciousness of health and the body. Because of the nature of correctional environments, however, parts of this continuum of care may be limited.

"Total institutions" and power, control and agency

One of the major barriers to encouraging public health promotion in correctional settings is the totality of the institutions. Goffman (1961) used the term "total institution" to describe settings that were characterized by closure to the outside world, the reconstruction of everyday living, an authoritarian bureaucratic organizational structure, and consequently a high degree of disciplinary control (Burns, 1992). Goffman describes the admission procedures as "systematic mortification" (mortification having the literal Latin meaning of "making dead"), a form of degradation ritual. This amounts to a custodial institution taking control over many aspects if its inmates' lives and removing any tolerable conception of self (Burns, 1992, pp. 148–149). Burns goes so far as to call this a "training in unfitness for the world outside," or a form of deculturation (p. 149).

This deterioration of the inmate's capacity for life on the outside, Burns argues, produces a diminished self, where inmates' self-image is kept under constant attack and forced into a submissive or suppliant role, with the emphasis on the lack of power to control their circumstances. Further, there may be a formal or arbitrary system of punishments for inmates who fail to adopt an appropriately submissive or deferential attitude toward authority (Burns, 1992, p. 52). The deprivation of liberty in a total institution may be accompanied by a deprivation of control of even the smallest and most personal aspects of human behavior, such as eating, sleeping and elimination.

The implications of the impact of a total institution on an individual's agency and self-esteem may be serious, especially as they relate to health behaviors. Where the autonomy of the self is systematically violated by what Goffman (1961, p. 38) calls "regimentation and tyrannisation," health may become just another battleground for power over the lives of inmates. While Goffman was writing of total institutions over 50 years ago, and in many jurisdictions the totality of the prison experience has not only subsided but in many cases has been systematically reduced in order to facilitate rehabilitation, it may still constitute a major barrier to health education. Thus, before any program is introduced into a correctional setting, we must determine the degree of "totality" of the institution, and if it is high in its control of the lives of inmates, whether a health education or promotion program can succeed if there is such domination over their lives and "role dispossession" (Goffman, 1961, p. 14) that their sense of agency has been irrevocably damaged. Even where the individual's agency to think and act in health matters is relatively undamaged, unless the institution's management is supportive of the introduction of health education and development programs, they are simply likely to become a source of tension over power and control, especially if they are seen as emancipating inmates. Thus, programs need to be firmly grounded in concrete health-improvement issues. Smith (2000) has noted that general principles such as health empowerment, positive health and health autonomy are vague. Where they can be grounded in self-generated health interests and concerns, and where they lead to exploration, understanding and mastery of individual and system-level health constraints, as in Freire's approach, they become specific outcomes for specific health concerns, rather than just general principles. Any programs in specific systems and institutions will require clear administrative buy-in.

Administrative concerns

However, increased screening and sensitization to health needs may have significant budgetary considerations. For example, increased screening for HIV or Hepatitis B will have implications for treatment provision for newly detected cases (treatment which is expensive and ongoing). Opposition to health literacy programs in correctional settings may arise from the potential cost of treatment rather than from issues of power and control.

A second administrative concern may relate to health education providing inmates with information which may be misused to simulate illness or to fake symptoms in order to obtain medication for oneself or for barter. This is a real concern which needs to be taken seriously. However, correctional settings may contain as many "jailhouse doctors" as "jailhouse lawyers" and it is unlikely that any information that is not already known by drug users, who are very knowledgeable about how to feign illness to obtain medication, will be provided. Further, most medications desired by inmates are analgesics and psychotropic medications, usually used to treat pain and psychiatric symptoms, respectively. They are inappropriate to treat all but a couple of the health issues that inmates listed in Table 6.1.

Conclusions

Prisoners and others in custodial care represent a group that is most in need of public health and health promotion interventions, given their social class and concomitant inmate culture and health issues. Senior and Shaw (2007, p. 393) note that

> When not in custody, prisoners often live chaotic lives characterized by offending, drug misuse, lack of engagement with normal societal

structures and impermanence in terms of accommodation and family relationships. These elements are then imported into prisons when people are in custody.

Such *importation* largely but not exclusively defines the health care issues within prison. The inmate may also be introduced to, or expand, some health risk behaviors while incarcerated. However, we also need to ask what elements may be *exported* back into the community by the released inmate. Prisons can play a part in providing peer health education into disadvantaged communities as well as appropriate health promotion and prevention services within the prison. Indeed, King and McDermott (1995) observe that prison may also focus the attention of the inmate on their health through being given time to dwell on their signs and symptoms. Freire's approach to education may provide both the model and the empowerment to not only develop the concept of a "healthy prison," but also to translate the concept of public health and disease prevention into disadvantaged free world communities, and at the same time to provide a sense of health emancipation and self worth, both as persons and as bodies, to inmates.

There are several policy implications that arise from this chapter. Prison health policies which engage in health education and promotion will not only have the potential to reduce some significant prison and free world health conditions and costs, but will also have equivalent effects in the wider community on re-entry both directly and through the peer-education influence of current and former inmates. Prison health education may also provide opportunities for facilitating inmates' empowerment in the context of their bodies and health. Using Freire's model to increase health literacy and promote healthy (or less risky) behaviors in inmates provides an opportunity to develop demonstration projects to empirically assess the individual, institutional and community-level impacts of such public health programs.

7 Prison staff occupational health and safety and its relationship with inmate health[1]

People sharing an environment, even with different patterns of social structure and movement, will also share many of the same health and environmental risks. In a prison or jail context, therefore, there may be significant overlap in risks – and health protective factors – between prisoners and prison staff. Thus, it makes no sense to consider the health needs of prisoners without realizing that in many instances they are closely connected with occupational health and safety issues of prison staff, and vice versa. In a close and closed community, infectious diseases will spread with little distinction between the inmates and the custodial staff. Further, where the environment is stressful, that stress will be manifested in both the inmates and the staff, and where it is unsafe, the lack of safety will extend to staff–prisoner as well as prisoner–prisoner interactions. In addition, environmental hazards will impact both staff and inmates, whether through cold, heat, noise, poor ventilation or environmental toxins such as asbestos or lead. Inmates and staff breathe the same air, walk in the same buildings, touch the same objects, and often suffer the same stresses of the psychological and physical environment. Sometimes they will eat food prepared in the same kitchens by the same staff or inmates. From a physical and psychological health perspective, if a prison is an unhealthy environment for inmates, it will also be unhealthy for staff. Thus, it makes no sense to consider the health needs of prisoners without realizing that in many instances they are closely connected with occupational health and safety needs of prison staff, and vice versa.

Prison staff as a neglected sector of occupational health

If prisoners can be considered a relatively forgotten sector of the community, prison staff might also be considered a relatively neglected sector of the workforce. The literature on the health and psychosocial stressors of correctional staff is sparse, and staff in correctional institutions are often considered in conjunction with other peace officers such as police, although the duties and risks may vary considerably (Hessl, 2001). Part of this confusion may lie in the fact that in some occupational databases, no distinction is made between police and correctional officers, and thus occupational and lifestyle hazards in the two groups cannot be separated. Further, as Jetté and Sidney (1991) observed, sometimes there is a traditionally adversarial relationship between management and unions where there is a suspicion of any form of testing of union members or their involvement in health-related or health-enhancement programs, and a wariness that information collected might not be in the best interests of their members. On the other hand, more recently other researchers have conducted large studies in correctional systems with a high degree of support and produced important findings that benefit both management and staff (Armstrong and Griffin, 2004; Alarid, 2009). All of these studies were carried out in North America, although they probably generalize to other Western correctional settings.

Long-term effects of correctional system work

Often, health issues of staff in the correctional system focus on short-term risks to health such as trauma or infectious diseases. The long-term effects of working in a correctional setting should also be considered: however, such studies rely on following up large samples of correctional staff over relatively long time periods, or looking at measures or markers of morbidity in correctional staff. Thus, they can be difficult and expensive, or depend on the availability of large state or national occupational data sets which distinguish correctional officers. When comparing mortality and morbidity by occupational category, Hessl (2001) notes that law enforcement personnel (police and corrections officers) have among the top ten proportional mortality (death) rates from ischemic heart disease (narrowing of the coronary arteries and decreased blood supply to the heart), with black officers having significantly higher rates than white officers. Hessl lists a number of health risks for correctional staff in the prison environment: tuberculosis; blood-borne pathogens (Hepatitis B and C, HIV) in injecting (or tattoo) equipment; lead and asbestos in old facilities; chemicals and solvents in prison industries; noise, heat and cold; the effect of shift work, including disordered sleep; trauma from violence; heightened risk of homicide or suicide; and, particularly, stress, which can lead to gastrointestinal complaints, an increased risk of heart disease, and alcohol abuse and subsequent cirrhosis of the liver.

Impact of stress

Stress is at the heart of the health issues confronting staff in prisons and other correctional institutions. To reiterate the point made at the beginning of this chapter, the health of prison staff and inmates is intertwined, particularly in the case of stress. Stressed prison staff produce stressed prisoners, and stressed prisoners produce stressed prison staff. The relationship can develop into a vicious cycle. It is thus in the interests of the health and safety of all concerned that the interdependence of prisoners and staff in prison health – infectious disease, violence, environmental hazards and stress – are seen to interact in a relatively closed system. I use the term "relatively" closed, because not only do prisoners get released, but prison staff return to the community at the end of their shifts, where the effects of disease and stress are transmitted to their families, with both immediate and long-term consequences.

Staff stress and prisoner stress interact

There are mutually dependent relationships between staff stress and prisoner stress, because both are caused by environmental conditions in the prison. Nurse *et al.* (2003) conducted focus groups of staff and prisoners separately at a medium-security prison in England and found that the key aspects of the prison environment that affected prisoners' mental health were isolation and lack of mental stimulation, which in turn encouraged drug misuse as a means of escape and to relieve mental tedium. All the prisoner focus groups emphasized the interactive nature of negative staff–prisoner relationships, where if an officer treated prisoners badly, prisoners would make that officer's life difficult, thus causing more stress for the officers. They also noted how fewer staff increased the amount of time prisoners spent in cells, which made prisoners more difficult to deal with, thus increasing stress levels of both staff and prisoners. Staff focus groups noted, in addition to the stress caused by increasing numbers of prisoners and its resultant increase in tensions between staff and inmates, problems arising from management style – lack of communication, insufficient information and lack of continuity of care with prisoners. Uniformed staff considered that stress was the most important issue affecting their health. Prison health care staff were also concerned about how other staff members would "offload their stress on them" (p. 482), as well as safety concerns about having to interview prisoners on their own in potentially unsafe situations. The pressure of increasing numbers of prisoners increased staff stress by decreasing the possibility of positive interactions with prisoners and the chance of identifying problems, with one staff member observing that "Only a couple of years ago there was enough time for staff to talk one on one with prisoners ... you could identify prisoners who were having problems" (p. 482). Such comments underscore the often interactive nature of relationships between staff and prisoners and their strong potential for contribution to stress in both groups.

Nurse *et al.*'s (2003) study found that stress differed between health care workers in prisons and uniformed officers. In an insightful study of nurses in English prisons, Walsh (2009) noted the cognitive dissonance often felt by nurses as a "care–custody conflict" created by the clash of the philosophies of caring and custody. This clash , argues Walsh, arises largely from the prison setting which has its focus on secure custody, while health care is often seen as secondary. She identifies this clash in her study of nurses working in prisons as "emotional labor," necessitating the nurses negotiating the web of demanding relationships that occur in health care in prisons. Such demands include ensuring that the prisoner feels confident in the nurse's ability or the prison officer feeling that the nurse understands the officer's perspective, or the prison's routine restricting the nurse's ability to provide particular or appropriate care. In Walsh's study, nurses also noted stresses inherent in managing aggression and manipulation, coping with prisoners whose offenses the nurses found it difficult to deal with emotionally, working alongside colleagues whose practice was felt to be substandard, and managing relationships with prison officer colleagues. Some described using detachment as a way of avoiding sympathy, empathy and care for prisoners. These data suggest that conflicting professional ideologies, combined with lack of any power in the prison structure, may take a higher toll in job-related stress on health care personnel in prisons.

A second stress-producing aspect of the job for corrections officers is the need to deal with violent and disruptive inmates (Parker, 2009). Parker designed and evaluated a training course for correctional officers in a "supermax" facility (designed for violent or disruptive inmates). The course was designed on the premise that the training that correctional staff had for dealing with such inmates, and in understanding mental health issues, was minimal. The ten-hour course was designed and taught by the National Alliance on Mental Illness especially for correctional staff, and focused on the specific conditions that correctional officers faced. Compared with the nine months before the course, incidents of assault by bodily waste (the so-called "prison officer cocktail") on officers by inmates in the unit after the course declined significantly to zero, and all incidents involving officers also significantly declined. Parker suggests that this was as a result of training correctional officers to better understand and deal with mentally ill offenders, including talking with offenders in a therapeutic manner, and working as an integral part of the mental health diagnosis and treatment process. This not only reduced violence against officers through providing officers with a better understanding of how to deal with the mentally disturbed, but also reduced the stress of working with difficult and potentially violent offenders. Thus, some workplace stressors are open to reduction through appropriate training and intervention programs. Further, Parker's data also confirm the close interactions between officers' adequacy of training and prisoners' behavior in stressful situations.

Organizational environment and stress

The prison physical and organizational environment itself may account for a considerable amount of stress and poor health in workers in the system – both correctional officers and correctional health and treatment personnel. In a landmark study of predictors of stress in both correctional officers and treatment personnel in the Arizona prison system, Armstrong and Griffin (2004) found that correctional officers and prison treatment staff scored similarly on measures of stress and on stress-related health problems (including headaches, fatigue and stomach trouble). High workplace stress (disturbance of physiological, psychological or social functioning in response to a condition in the work environment which poses a threat to well-being or safety) is experienced by large numbers of correctional staff (39 percent according to Lindquist and Whitehead in their 1986 study) and may be associated with a combination of factors such as the correctional environment itself and low pay and lack of benefits. One of the results of these high stressors is high staff turnover rates.

One of the organizational factors suggested by Armstrong and Griffin (2004) leading to stress is the shift in the United States from seeing correctional institutions as rehabilitative to a shift to seeing them as primarily punitive. This leads to a lack of clarity about role, job objectives and responsibilities, lack of support from superiors and lack of consistency in instructions and supervision.

Physical environment

Physical environment also constitutes a health and safety risk, with prison officers ranking second only to police officers in the number of workplace non-fatal violent incidents. Prison officers frequently perceive a constant threat of danger from those they supervise, with the suggestion that the threats are higher in maximum-security institutions. This is consistent with reports of higher rates of illness in prison officers in maximum-security prisons compared with minimum security ones (Armstrong and Griffin, 2004). However, the risk of physical danger is significantly higher to prison officers than to treatment staff, and so the finding of Armstrong and Griffin that there were no differences between the two groups in job stress and stress-related health conditions raises questions of the specific weighting of environmental stress on stress and health outcomes. They found that the strongest predictors of job stress for prison staff were role problems (conflict over differing and ambiguous job demands), but lack of intrinsic rewards, co-worker support and organizational support, and environmental safety were other significant contributors. For treatment staff, the findings were essentially similar.

For stress-related health problems, role problems again were strong predictors of physical symptoms, along with lack of organizational support. Interestingly, for treatment personnel, and to a lesser extent for prison officers, a second strong predictor of health problems was lack of intrinsic rewards on the job, while environmental safety also acted as a predictor of health problems for prison officers. As might be anticipated, demographic variables such as female gender, younger age and duration of employment in the prison system were also associated with increases in stress and health problems. These data, which have the additional strength of being based on a large sample of the total state correctional facility staff, confirm the anticipated linkages of stress and stress-related health problems, but point to management issues such as job role problems and lack of organizational support (and the presence or absence of intrinsic rewards in the job) as being of equal or greater import than environmental safety in predicting stress and stress-related health problems. The clear implication of these findings is that management issues may be of equal or greater significance than anticipated prisoner violence in the production of stress-related illness such as headaches, fatigue and stomach upsets. Armstrong and Griffin (2004) conclude that apart from perceptions of personal safety, sources of stress (as well as protective factors against stress) were similar in both custodial and treatment staff groups, with environmental factors having the strongest impacts.

Predictors of workplace stress and poor health

A study by Ogińska-Bulik (2005) among uniformed personnel in Poland, including a large sample of prison officers, suggests that the predictors of workplace stress have commonalities in prison officers across western cultures. As in most other work on workplace stress, Ogińska-Bulik (2005) used measures of stress-related illnesses (somatic complaints, anxiety and insomnia, social functioning disorders and symptoms of depression). She found that the lowest level of stress, the highest degree of a sense of social coherence and the highest degree of social support (along with the best health status) was found in prison officers, in comparison with the other uniformed servicemen (police, firefighters, security guards, city guards) . She also found, as did research in the United States and UK, that the best predictors of health status were stress at work and amount of social support. Thus, high workplace stress is associated with poorer health, and good social supports help to both reduce stress at work and are also associated with better health. Her data suggest that the predictors of workplace stress have commonalities in prison officers across western cultures, although the actual levels may depend on particular prison organizational and physical environments: thus, the level of stress compared with other uniformed professions may vary between and within countries.

Blood-borne disease

Taking an apparently very different health-related issue in prison staff, the risk of contracting blood-borne infectious diseases such as HIV, the findings are surprisingly similar in locating the problem in contextual rather than individual factors. Alarid (2009) carried out a study of nearly 200 correctional officers in a US Midwestern state and found that it was institutional variables rather than individual behavior that predicted exposure to HIV. It is important to note that HIV here serves as an exemplar infectious disease, since it is transmitted through blood and other body fluids, as are Hepatitis B and C, both very prevalent in prison populations, and both an order of magnitude more infectious than HIV (and with severe or potentially fatal consequences). Alarid notes that prison staff are likely to be first responders to physical altercations, accidents, medical emergencies and unpredictable and often hostile situations where sharp objects and body fluids may present risks. In addition, prison staff may frequently come into contact with needles discarded by inmates who don't have access to needle exchange or drug treatment, or from prison tattooing practices. She notes that a number of institutional variables are likely to increase risk, including higher prisoner-security-level units, afternoon and evening shifts when there is more misconduct on the part of prisoners, and length of time employed in the correctional system.

Alarid's data confirm that it is these institutional variables that are the best predictors of occupational exposure to blood-borne pathogens such as HIV. Custody level of inmates (a measure of the level of violence), length of employment (a measure of the cumulative level of exposure to risk situations) and rank (rank reflects the risk of being called to medical emergencies and altercations) all predicted level of exposure to blood-borne pathogens. Interestingly, for prisoner variables that impacted custodial staff risk of exposure, gender of prisoners was not a significant risk, but prisoner behavior (injecting drug use, tattooing, security level and inmate–inmate sex [for males]) all presented the greatest risk of HIV infection and thus the greatest potential threat to prison staff. What is important to note in both Armstrong and Griffin's and Alarid's work is that institutional and organizational variables may be strongly associated with health status or risks in correctional settings. Even where infectious agents such as HIV and Hepatitis B and C are involved, which are obviously dependent on their prevalence in the inmate population and the level of risk of needle sticks or other exposures to inmate blood and other body fluids, institutional factors also influence who is likely to be most at risk in the prison staff. Health of prison staff, therefore, needs to be understood not only from the immediate risk situation, but also from the perspective of the organizational and institutional factors that focus that risk, and which create the stressors that are associated with chronic disease.

Inmate and prison staff health interactions

Taken together, these data suggest that there is a close correspondence between the health of inmates and of prison staff, and that prison environmental and organizational issues may also play a significant role in the health, particularly the long-term health, of custodial staff. Interestingly, the pattern also holds with blood-borne infectious diseases, suggesting that the concept of risk environments, as much as risk sources and behaviors, needs to be considered. In particular, long-term health consequences of working in a custodial environment (and the role of stress and environment) need to be better studied. However, any distinction between inmate health and custodial staff health, either short-term or long-term, is likely to be arbitrary, and the concept of a healthy prison needs to embrace both inmate and staff health as integral to one another.

8 Ensuring health in prison and achieving healthy prisons

The TECH model[1]

In 1995 the World Health Organization (WHO)/Europe first launched the "Health in Prisons" project (Møller et al., 2007). More recently, the WHO published "Health in Prisons," a document that summarizes the philosophy and practice of a "whole-prison approach" toward achieving health in prisons. "Health in prison" is the process of *providing* comprehensive health services and education in prison. "*Achieving a healthy prison*" (Møller et al., 2007, p. 2) is the *long-term goal* of achieving a sustainable, health-promoting prison. "Health in prison" represents and results from the provision of comprehensive health services and education to prisoners. A "healthy prison" extends this concept and is understood as the achievement and long-term maintenance of a prison that promotes the health of both inmates *and* correctional staff while in prison and as they interface with the community.

The concept of the "healthy prison" represents a complete transformation of the "total prison" concept. In a total prison, the organization, regime and physical prison structure are dedicated to punishment, to making prison a profoundly negative experience that would serve as a deterrent to crime. The healthy prison, on the other hand, is the product of an environment that, within the confines of the law and the penal system, promotes and maintains health. Møller et al. use the terms "health promoting prison" and "whole-prison approach" to describe such a system, and note that "sustainability" is the characteristic of achieving a healthy prison (2007, p. 1). The health of the whole prison must be considered – that of both staff and inmates – as well as the environment (including occupational health and safety). The *process* of achieving a healthy prison, however, particularly in resource-poor areas, has not been clearly addressed, and this chapter attempts to provide an appropriate and simple process model based on risk-reduction models. We extend Møller et al.'s point that countries with basic or rudimentary services will need support to introduce the changes that are described in "Health in Prisons." That is, we argue that even in settings with minimal or no economic resources, there are still actions that can be taken that can reduce health risks and improve health. There are, however, no good process models to guide prison administrators and staff through such a course of action, and this chapter attempts to provide such a model.

Health in prison: the WHO model

The WHO Health in Prisons project (Møller *et al.*, 2007) introduced the concept of health in prisons or health-promoting prisons. This latter phrase covers prisons in which

> The risks to health are reduced to a minimum; essential prison duties such as maintenance of security are undertaken in a caring atmosphere that recognizes the inherent dignity of every prisoner and their human rights; health services are provided to the level and in a professional manner equivalent to what is provided in the country as a whole; and a whole-prison approach to promoting health and welfare is the norm.
>
> (p. xvi)

Møller *et al.* (2007) list the essential steps in setting up health in prisons. First, all staff must be involved, including the senior management who determine the prison climate. Second, it must be sustainable, which will involve creating strong links between prison health care services and the health services of the local community. These essential components thus involve buy-in at a political level, by management, by staff, by prisoners, and by the local community health system.

The emphasis on a healthy prison arises from the recognition that "prison service is a public service" (Møller *et al.*, 2007, p. 2). Møller *et al.* emphasize that good prison health is essential to good public health. From the community perspective, in turn, there needs to be a recognition that the opportunities presented by a prison are substantial and potentially cost-effective, by allowing access to people who are at high medical risk and high socioeconomic disadvantage, and who are often very difficult to reach in terms of locating them and in terms of expense and staff time while out in the community. The movement of people already infected, or at high disease risk, into correctional environments and back into society without effective treatment or follow-up, or indeed preventive education, gives rise to the spread of diseases inside the system and beyond it. Finally, they emphasize that the physical conditions in many prisons are unhealthy. This will largely depend on the living conditions in prisons, which are usually better in most developed countries, and usually worse in less-developed, resource-poor settings. While in the latter case these may be beyond the control of management and staff or require political buy-in, issues may include overcrowding, violence, lack of fresh air, lack of light, poor food and water quality, poor sanitation, and infection-spreading activities such as tattooing, use (including injecting) of drugs and sexual activity (sometimes coerced) without the availability of protection from STIs and HIV. Møller *et al.* (2007) thus provide a crucial philosophical and practical starting point for thinking about health in prisons.

Healthy settings

The WHO has also pioneered the concept of "healthy settings" – perhaps best known by the "healthy cities" movement (Harpham *et al.*, 2001). Such setting-based approaches are characterized by "a holistic and multi-disciplinary method which integrates action across risk factors. The goal is to maximize disease prevention via a 'whole system approach'," which has its roots in the Ottawa charter of 1986 (WHO, n.d.). Using this model, we believe that prisons can also benefit from being seen as potentially "healthy settings": healthy prisons, which integrate actions from multiple health processes into a setting approach, and move beyond healthy individuals.

From health in prisons to achieving healthy prisons

This conceptual transformation to a "healthy prison" as a setting can only come about by rethinking or reshaping to some degree the concept of the prison and the prisoner. First, it requires that we see the prison not as an environment totally closed to the outside world, but almost completely open. It is open in the temporal sense, in that most prisoners will move in and out – and, given recidivism rates, possibly several times – for time-limited stays. It becomes, in modern usage, a place of *behavioral* quarantine (to remove the prisoner from endangering the free world) as well as punishment by the deprivation of liberty. It is open in the sense of the transmission of infectious organisms between prisoners and prison staff, prisoners and visitors and prisoners and the community – both in terms of what they bring in, and what they take out on release. In *health* terms, then, it may be less of a quarantine –and may be more akin to an incubator and/or a vector of disease, where overcrowding and risky practices may multiply risk.

Second, the healthy prison requires that the prisoner be seen as more than a space-occupying body, but as a functioning body, in both the physical and mental sense. The prisoner moves from being an object of detention to a body with medical and mental health care needs: that is, they move from the simple legal status of a body legally detained and subject to judicial control, to a body to be treated and health maintained or improved. In some ways, this parallels the move from prison as a place of incarceration to a place of correction – which is the intention behind the reference to the prison system as a "correctional system," even if there is often little formal attention to rehabilitation or "correction."

Third, to extend this idea further, a healthy prison recognizes that there has been a shift from the "total prisoner" toward the "total patient," where the focus is on the inmate as a potentially healthy body rather than just a correctional entity. The total patient prisoner, as opposed to the penal prisoner, exists with risk behaviors and in an environment that may often promote poor health. This is a conundrum: in an environment which is often physically drab and intellectually boring, illicit behaviors like smoking, drug use and alcohol consumption become adaptations for stimulation and entertainment. Here, the conflict between prisoner and patient becomes most salient, where the punitive and the curative or preventive aspects of prison may collide. The concept of the healthy prison is an attempt to integrate the penal and the medical in the persons of the prisoners and the custodial staff, both of whom have a right to a healthy and safe prison environment.

Healthy prisons as restorative justice

However, there need not be a tension between the two. Indeed, the criminological concept of restorative justice might be extended to prison health care. Restorative justice involves, in addition to making amends, a broader function of the restoration into safe communities of offenders (Duff, 2003). If we see the concept of restorative justice in the sense of the wider community, then part of the correctional process is to return the released inmate *restored* in whatever sense can benefit the community – possessing work-related skills, with substance abuse treated and mental health problems stabilized, and with health issues that might cost the community directly or indirectly treated or prevented. In this sense of restorative justice, the restoration is to the community and not specifically just to the victim. We must also consider the simultaneous provision of appropriate occupational health care to prison staff as part of a "restoration" by recompense for the difficult and sometimes dangerous working conditions that exist in prisons. A healthy prison, therefore, should be seen as an integral part of the concept of restorative justice as much as an integral part of the concept of public health. Viewed through the lens of restorative justice, the healthy prison is one where the aims of criminal justice and public health intersect.

Finally, classically, prisons have been institutions developed not only for punishment but also for the protection of the community. As Møller *et al.* (2007) argue, healthy prisons are completely consistent with this aspect of criminology: the risks they protect the community from include infectious diseases, the effects of drug and alcohol use and violence, plus the longer-term costs of preventable disease. Protection involves several distinct aspects of medicine. Initially, prisoners who have missed important routine vaccinations previously should receive those vaccinations where medically appropriate, in a process of making good any deficits that may have occurred in population coverage. In addition, they should/can be vaccinated against conditions which are prevalent in prisons, such as Hepatitis B, and pneumococcal infections, for protection both of the free world and of the prison communities. For juvenile offenders, human papillomavirus (HPV) vaccinations might also be considered, given their high level of sexual risk behavior. Then, existing symptomatic problems need to be treated according to standard medical practice. In resource-limited settings, non-urgent and elective conditions may need to be scheduled as conditions and resources permit. Lastly, bearing in mind that the great majority of inmates will return to the community, communities need to be protected against future dangers that released inmates may present. This includes not only specific risks of infections associated with drug and sexual risk behaviors (e.g., HIV, STIs, Hepatitis B and C, HPV) and violence, but also so-called "victimless" health behavior deficits that do indeed have victims (the individual), but more importantly pose health costs to the community, such as smoking, obesity, diabetes and other chronic conditions linked to lifestyle (Elliott, 2007; Binswanger *et al.*, 2009; Harzke *et al.*, 2010). Put simply, prison health programs may not only be restorative in reducing the inmate's risk to the community, but they also play an important role in reducing the health-related cost to the community of the returning inmate as regards both infectious and longer-term chronic diseases. The community is protected through the implementation of behavioral risk-reduction interventions to decrease the probability of drug-related and violent crime that result from addiction to drugs and alcohol and problems with anger and impulse management – treatable mental and physical health-related issues. It is a logical extension to move one small step further to protect the community from other preventable health-related conditions.

Achieving healthy prisons: the TECH model

Achieving healthy prisons may be easier in more developed countries and penal systems than in resource-poor settings and in less-developed countries. It is important for us to develop a model that is equally applicable in systems with relatively high and low or no resources for health, rather than simply in better-resourced areas. We present the TECH model as one approach to achieving healthy prisons, which describes health-promoting activities in four domains, and from immediate acute conditions to longer-term maintenance. It is designed to be applicable to low- as well as high-resource settings, and is based on a risk-reduction model: that is, in any setting, there will still be some risk-reducing activities or interventions that are possible.

Faced with scarce financial resources and often political disinterest, how can correctional facilities move toward healthy prisons? The TECH model provides a series of steps to develop healthy prisons. TECH is the acronym referring (see Table 8.1) to the four domains: **T** (Test and treat infectious diseases and provide vaccinations, if available); **E** (Environmental modification to reduce risks); **C** (Control of chronic diseases); and **H** (Health maintenance and health education). While the TECH model is presented sequentially, these steps do not necessarily need to be followed in order, although it starts with the more urgent health needs and moves to the maintenance of health. It can be "high TECH," in that it is implemented in some detail across all domains, or "low TECH," where it is implemented on an as-possible basis or where only the low- or no-cost domains are implemented.

Table 8.1 Healthy prisons domain: the TECH model

---

*T*est and treat infectious diseases
- Identify and treat infectious diseases
- Vaccinate if any childhood or routine vaccines were missed
- Vaccinate for high-risk prison diseases where possible (e.g., Hepatitis B, pneumococcus)

*E*nvironmental modification to prevent disease transmission
- Identify and remove vectors (e.g., insects, sanitary arrangements)
- Identify inmate–inmate and inmate–staff transmission possibilities and attempt to control these
- Identify unhealthy environmental factors (e.g., smoking, lack of exercise, food) and modify as much as possible

*C*hronic disease identification and treatment
- Screen for chronic diseases
- Treat where possible (e.g., blood pressure, diabetes, asthma)
- Consider prevention programs

*H*ealth maintenance and education
- Screen and treat incoming inmates and staff
- Educate inmates and staff about health, safety and self-maintenance of health
- Maintain inmate health and staff health peer-education systems if possible

---

In some cases, political and employee pressures will make the development of a healthy environment for *staff* an easier place to start than with inmate treatment. In others, legal decisions, such as *Coleman/Plata* v. *Schwarzenegger* in California, will prioritize and mandate improving *inmate* health and treatment. In *Coleman/Plata* v. *Schwarzenegger*, the state of California was ordered to release 34,000 prisoners of the state total of nearly 150,000 because health conditions in the state prisons were considered unacceptable. The magnitude and impact of this remedy underscores the fact that health issues in prisons are taken very seriously by the courts in many jurisdictions. However, given the interactions between inmate and staff health, it makes no sense to limit health issues to just inmates or just staff: both groups should be screened and treated within the same time frame to avoid cross-infection or cross-impact of negative environmental conditions between groups (Ross, 2010).

Treat infectious diseases

First, existing infectious diseases need to be identified and treated. These will usually include, but are not limited to: tuberculosis, STIs such as syphilis, gonorrhea and Chlamydia, HIV, Hepatitis B and C, particularly where injecting drug users make up a significant part of the prison population. Rates of infection can vary enormously between jurisdictions. Rodriguez *et al.* (2002) report Hepatitis C rates in the city of Ciudad Juárez, Mexico at

100 percent of prisoners, while over the border in Texas, Baillargeon *et al.* (2003) report male rates as being 27 percent and female rates as 35 percent (state jails) to 48 percent (state prisons). Tuberculosis rates can vary from about half the country's new cases occurring in prison in Russia (Coninx *et al.*, 2000), to being a rare event in Scandinavian countries.

In tropical areas and where prevalent, Hansen's disease (leprosy), malaria and other parasitic diseases such as schistosomiasis, lymphatic filariasis and onchocerciasis (which are easily treatable) should also be identified and treated. Second, inmates are often at risk of having missed routine childhood vaccinations, and where medically appropriate, these should be given. However, for some childhood vaccinations, the individual subsequently may have become immune by exposure to the disease (e.g., Hepatitis A) and not need vaccination. State requirements for vaccinations vary from state to state and country to country and local recommendations must be checked. State, county and city public health departments can advise on the most important local requirements. However, common vaccinations in childhood may include diphtheria, tetanus, pertussis (whooping cough), measles, mumps, rubella, varicella (chickenpox), meningococcus and Hepatitis A. While these may not seem important to adults, we need to bear in mind that transmission to visitors (including children), and from prison staff to their families, may have serious or fatal consequences to people outside the prison (particularly the young and the old), and that vaccination is part of community protection for diseases, which are no respecters of walls or segregation. For vaccination and the consequences of lack of vaccination, prisons must be recognized as an integral part of the community.

Third, there are diseases that are likely to be prevalent in prison populations and which, if untreated, may be associated with increased transmission in prison, and where vaccination as a preventive measure may need to be considered. Those most likely to impact prison populations and workers include Hepatitis B and pneumococcus (bacteria causing pneumococcal pneumonia, and possibly blood, lung, middle ear and nervous infection). In areas with high levels of tuberculosis transmission, BCG vaccination may also need to be considered if people have not already been vaccinated. Tuberculosis in prison populations may be 10–100 times the rate in local populations and exacerbated by overcrowding, heavy smoking, poor nutrition and HIV infection (Møller *et al.*, 2007).

In all these cases, an understanding of local population rates of disease, and specifically infection and susceptibility rates among inmates and staff who have direct prisoner contact, must be considered before making any recommendations. Finally, any vaccination program should be carried out in close collaboration with a national or local health department to ensure the vaccinations are appropriate to local risk and need. Because vaccination costs are covered by the government in many countries, this should also reduce cost to the prison.

Environmental modification to prevent disease transmission

First, identify vectors of transmission from disease reservoir to host. These may include insect vectors, such as mosquitoes, which may transmit malaria or other infectious diseases. Simple precautions such as spraying or removing standing water which may be breeding areas for mosquitoes in the prison surrounds can be effective. In Central and South America, Chagas disease is a serious and sometimes fatal condition transmitted by the reduviid insect. Spider or other insect bites may cause discomfort and provide an opportunity for infection by *Staphylococci* or other bacteria. What are commonly referred to as "spider bites" in North American prisons are usually Staphylococcal infections rather than arachnid bites. Proper ventilation and sunlight can reduce the transmission of tuberculosis (Madhukar *et al.*, 2006).

Second, survey transmission possibilities and see which can be easily modified in the prison environment. Many of these will already be subject to investigation, such as identifying and removing illegal tattooing equipment and illegal needles and syringes for injecting drugs. Paradoxically, sometimes removing injecting equipment may mean that undetected injecting equipment is spread among even more inmates, increasing rather than decreasing the risk. Some countries (including Switzerland, Germany, Spain, Moldova, Kyrgyzstan, Belarus and Armenia) have already successfully introduced needle and syringe exchange programs in their prisons (Elliott, 2007). As an alternative, providing bleach to clean previously used injection or tattoo equipment is a cheap and viable risk reduction. Such programs will have benefits for staff by decreasing the potential for infection through needlestick injury during searches (or other incidents).

Because both consensual and non-consensual sexual behavior occurs in prisons at varying levels, condom provision and use is another successful environmental intervention (Dolan *et al.*, 2004; WHO, 2007). Rape prevention programs in prisons also make use of environmental modifications, including segregation of juvenile and first-time offenders from more experienced or violent inmates, removing prisoners from dorms to rooms, and moving from the row to the pod design to enable better supervision of inmates as well as changes in prison culture (National Institute of Justice, 2008).

Third, other environmental interventions will have significant impacts on health. Banning smoking in prison units can have a major immediate and longer-term impact on health. Improvement of food and nutrition can also improve inmate health and is not necessarily more expensive. It may require specific retraining for catering management and staff, but if this occurs as job training, it can be considered an occupational benefit rather than a burden. For inmates who are responsible for food preparation, such additional training may have occupational benefits for them post-release. Depending on space and security availability, provision of more exercise time or equipment may have significant physical health benefits as well as mental health benefits.

Environmental modifications that are related to changes or extensions in the prison structure will prove much more expensive but should be considered in longer-term planning. Overcrowding has both direct and indirect health consequences and may be considered a violation of human or constitutional rights, as suggested by the recent Californian decision in *Coleman/Plata* v. *Schwarzenegger* by the US judiciary. Sanitation is a second area that has potential health consequences. Use of "slopping out" (in-cell bucket sanitation and its regular emptying) has very high potential for disease transmission of Hepatitis A and other infectious diseases, particularly dysentery caused by *Giardia*, *Shigella* and *Clostridium*. While very rare, fatal epidemics such as typhoid and cholera are also spread by this route. Bear in mind that some people may be carriers of these diseases without showing symptoms, such that absence of disease symptoms does not necessarily indicate that the disease is not being transmitted. Partial minimization of risk in "slopping out" might include reducing the distance (and chance of spillage) that waste is carried, limiting the number of people potentially exposed to waste and promoting cheap and simple but very effective precautions, such as thorough hand-washing after slopping-out. While "slopping out" is increasingly rare in western Europe, the United States and Canada, it is still common in much of the less-developed world.

Chronic disease identification and treatment

The prevalence of several non-infectious chronic diseases in prison populations, especially those with significant proportions of inmates over the age of 30 years, appears to be similar to or exceed that of the local non-incarcerated population in the United States (Harzke *et al.*, 2010; Wilper *et al.*, 2009; Binswanger *et al.*, 2009). These conditions include but are not limited to hypertension, diabetes, asthma, cardiovascular disease and liver disease. The prevalence and progression of these conditions are associated with aging, and all require regular clinical monitoring and/or daily pharmacologic management. However, for most of these conditions, treatments are generic and relatively low-cost, and all of these conditions may also be improved through proper nutrition, increased exercise, decreased BMI and/or improved environmental conditions in the prison context (e.g., improved air quality). Non-medical interventions such as exercise and weight-loss programs are low-cost and effective in reducing disease progression or development of disease. An exception may be alcoholic liver disease, which often co-occurs with and is exacerbated by Hepatitis B or C, the treatment of which may be outside the range of economic possibilities for many prisons where health budgets are limited, even in more developed countries. Psychiatric disorders and chronic mental health issues are highly prevalent in prison populations. In a systematic review of 62 studies of serious mental disorders in prison populations from 12 countries, Fazel and Danesh (2002) estimated that 3.7 percent of incarcerated or detained men had a psychotic illness, 10 percent had major depression and 65 percent had a personality disorder; women showed similar prevalence of depression (12 percent) and psychotic disorders (4 percent) and lower estimated prevalence of personality disorder (42 percent). On the basis of this study, the prevalence of serious mental disorders appears to vary considerably across countries, both overall and by gender, but is consistently higher in prison populations than in the local, non-incarcerated population. Mental health problems may be exacerbated by detention, especially if undiagnosed and untreated or under-treated. Prisoners with major psychiatric disorders (e.g., major depressive disorder, bipolar disorder, schizophrenia or other psychotic disorder) demonstrate higher rates of suicide in prison (Baillargeon *et al.* 2009b; Fazel *et al.*, 2008). Prisoners with major psychiatric disorders have substantially increased risk of multiple incarcerations (Baillargeon *et al.*, 2009a), suggesting that, even when treated in the prison setting, many prisoners are not receiving adequate mental health care in the community after release. Although mental health care of prisoners varies widely across countries and across jurisdictions, recommendations from developed countries suggest that mental health screening by qualified professionals and treatment with appropriate psychotropic medications should be provided when possible (NCCHC, 2008). That is, as with any chronic disease, initial screening and ongoing treatment are necessary.

Although prevalence estimates of substance abuse and dependence vary widely across prison populations, this special subset of psychiatric disorders is also highly prevalent in prison populations, typically many orders of magnitude higher than the local general population. In a systematic review of 13 studies representing four developed countries (England, Ireland, New Zealand and the United States), prevalence estimates of alcohol abuse or dependence ranged from 18 percent to 40 percent in male prisoners and from 10 percent to 24 percent in female prisoners. In this same review, prevalence estimates of substance use or dependence (excluding alcohol) ranged from 10 percent to 48 percent in male prisoners and from 30 percent to 60 percent in female prisoners. Offenders with substance use issues are more likely to be re-arrested and re-incarcerated (National Center on Addiction and Substance Abuse, 2010). Moreover, offenders who have substance use disorders co-occurring with other psychiatric disorders are substantially more likely to be reincarcerated than those with substance use disorders or psychiatric disorders alone (Baillargeon *et al.*, 2010). As with other chronic conditions, it is recommended that prisoners are screened and treated for substance abuse and dependence. Treatment plans should be comprehensive, individualized and evidence based. For example, prison-based therapeutic communities combined with aftercare (post-release) has been consistently shown as effective in reducing relapse and recidivism

(Mullen *et al.*, 2001; Wexler *et al.*, 1999; Martin *et al.*, 1999). Treatment may also include pharmacologic intervention. Provision of methadone maintenance for opiate addicts in prisons pre-release has been routine in some prison systems for several decades. Dolan *et al.* (1996) evaluated the methadone maintenance program in New South Wales (Australia) prisons, where it was introduced in 1987, and found that volunteer methadone maintenance is associated with reduced injecting in prisons. More recently, Kinlock *et al.* (2008) conducted a randomized trial in the United States and found that compared with counseling alone, or counseling with the chance of commencing methadone maintenance on release, starting methadone maintenance in prison led to participants being more likely to attend drug treatment, less likely to report heroin or cocaine use or criminal activity post-release, and less likely to be re-incarcerated. Methadone maintenance in prisons has been widely accepted in a number of jurisdictions and its benefits in reducing injecting in prison, relapse on release, and re-offending has been clearly demonstrated.

Health maintenance and health education

Health maintenance seeks to continue the state of health that has been achieved through the previous (T, E, C) stages of developing healthy prisons. This requires continuing to screen and treat inmates on admission for chronic health conditions and infectious diseases, to maintain the health of the prison. It requires maintenance of health-promotion efforts in the prison, whether the peer education programs or the interventions such as diet, exercise, weight loss, smoking or drug cessation, and maintaining hand-washing and reducing environmental risks (including for infectious diseases and disease vectors such as mosquitoes and other insects). It also includes considering modifications to the fabric or structure of the prison in the light of health-related concerns.

Treatment is important, but the number of cases will continue to grow if maintenance of chronic and prevention of acute conditions does not occur. If there is no maintenance of health, re-treatment will be required, which is more costly than maintenance or prevention. Maintenance also has the function of education and training peer educators (both inmates and staff) to maintain accurate health information transmission both inside and outside the prison (Ross, 2011).

Finally, education of inmates and staff needs to occur on a regular basis. The frequency of this will, to a large extent, depend on the rate of inmate and staff turnover in a prison. With shorter sentences and faster turnover, education needs to be repeated more often. In systems with peer education programs, the frequency of peer educator training must be frequent enough to maintain a critical mass of peer educators. Peer education is crucial in translating the health education from a prison to a community context, since inmate peer educators will on release become informal community peer educators. They also have the advantage of providing education within the appropriate cultural and language limitations. In addition, much health education takes place in informal settings and in social interaction, and here peer educators are particularly valuable (Ross *et al.*, 2006). In resource-poor settings, training trainers as peer educators may be an excellent way of widely disseminating health education.

Conclusions

Focusing on health in prisons is a process that leads to development of healthy prisons. The cornerstone for health in prisons is the WHO *Health in Prisons* guide (Møller *et al.*, 2007), which has as its goal health in prisons. However, the concept of a "healthy prison" goes beyond this, to describe a prison as a setting where the health of inmates and staff is a recognized – and implemented – goal of the institution. However, there are no good process models which provide an indication of how to achieve a healthy prison. Further, most research on health in prisons refers to institutions in the developed world. Nor are there good criteria for judging prison health outcomes. It is important to provide a model which is realistic to implement in part or in whole in prisons in less developed countries, and in very resource-poor settings. While it will be difficult to provide good health in prisons in such settings, there are nevertheless a number of steps that can be taken at low or no cost, and in collaboration with local health efforts, which can improve prison health for both inmates and staff.

It is important to locate health in prisons as part of a restorative justice approach, where inmates returning to the community come back relatively healthy and not as a drain on community resources. It is further important to recognize that a healthy prison workplace for prison staff can only be achieved if it is also healthy for inmates. The role of prison staff in promoting healthy prisons rests on their buy-in to the concept and recognition that a healthy prison is a benefit for themselves and their families as well. Without staff support, attempts to create healthy prisons are unlikely to succeed.

Thus, we have designed the TECH model to describe the steps that can be taken to promote health in prisons and lead to healthy prisons. TECH is the acronym referring (see Table 8.1) to the four domains: *T* (Test and treat infectious diseases and provide vaccinations, if available); *E* (Environmental modification to reduce risks); *C* (Control of chronic diseases); and *H* (Health maintenance and health education). It can be "high TECH" or "low TECH," depending on settings and resources. "High TECH" implementation will involve greater cost and outlay of resources, whereas "low TECH" may cover only a few domains, involve some staff time and energy, but can be achieved at minimal cost. There is, we hope, some provision for the TECH model to be implemented in all levels of prisons, from the institution which provides comprehensive medical and health services, to the institution which has no health services and relies on referral to a local hospital for serious cases. Taking a comprehensive approach to achieving healthy prisons that is applicable internationally and across levels of available resources by providing this four-domain model is a first step in characterizing the components of a healthy prison and the processes to achieve this.

9 Mental health and treatment in prisons

Hospitals of last resort or rehabilitation?

Mental health issues and prison health are heavily inter-dependent issues. The nature of the incarcerated population makes it likely that in some areas – for example, personality disorders where criminal activity is one of the defining characteristics of the disorder – there will be considerable overlap. From a public health point of view, screening for major mental disorders in prisons is crucial. While the more spectacular and serious disorders will often be selected out at the level of the court by diverting those who are considered unfit to plead by reason of mental illness to special facilities for the "criminally insane," prisons may still have to deal with those with serious mental illness who are not diverted. For this reason prisons have sometimes been referred to as "hospitals of last resort."

There is also the issue of incarcerogenic mental health – that where the prison or other custodial environment *causes or exacerbates* mental health problems – to consider. This can range from generating distress, or exacerbating existing, psychological problems to the extreme of attempted or completed suicides in prison.

Antisocial personality disorder

By its nature and the fact that people with these disorders are more likely to come to the attention of the authorities, antisocial personality disorder is frequently seen in prison settings. The *Diagnostic and Statistical Manual of the American Psychiatric Association* (DSM IV-TR) describes this as

> A pervasive pattern of disregard for and violation of the rights of others occurring since age 15 years, as indicated by three or more of the following:
>
> 1 failure to conform to social norms with respect to lawful behaviors as indicated by repeatedly performing acts that are grounds for arrest;
> 2 deception, as indicated by repeatedly lying, use of aliases, or conning others for personal profit or pleasure;

3   impulsiveness or failure to plan ahead;
4   irritability and aggressiveness, as indicated by repeated physical fights or assaults;
5   reckless disregard for safety of self or others;
6   consistent irresponsibility, as indicated by repeated failure to sustain consistent work behavior or honor financial obligations;
7   lack of remorse, as indicated by being indifferent to or rationalizing having hurt, mistreated or stolen from another.

The parallel definition by the WHO's International Classification of Diseases (ICD-10) defines a very similar category, "dissocial personality disorder," characterized by at least three of the following:

1   Callous unconcern for the feelings of others;
2   gross and persistent attitude of irresponsibility and disregard for social norms, rules and obligations;
3   incapacity to maintain enduring relationships, though having no difficulty in establishing them;
4   very low tolerance to frustration and a low threshold for discharge of aggression, including violence;
5   incapacity to experience guilt or to profit from experience, particularly punishment;
6   Markedly prone to blame others or to offer plausible rationalizations for the behavior that has brought the person into conflict with society.

Both of these definitions emphasize behavior that is likely to dramatically enhance the chances of being imprisoned. The epidemiology of antisocial personality disorder (Fazel and Danesh, 2002), based on a summary of over 60 studies, consistently shows that it is more likely to be seen in male than female prisoners, and that 47 percent of male prisoners and 21 percent of female prisoners meet the criteria for this diagnosis. It is clearly the most common mental health diagnosis that prison staff are likely to meet. Treatment, however, is less clear-cut. Fisher and O'Donohue (2006) suggest that contingency management programs (or other reward systems) may be moderately useful for people with antisocial personality disorders. However, this is likely to be more useful for *management* in a prison setting than as a long-term treatment, even if prison staff have the levels of staffing and training to deal with antisocial/dissocial personality disorder (which is unlikely in many settings).

Serious mental illness in prisons

The proportion of offenders in prisons who have serious mental illness appears to be relatively constant. Magaletta *et al.* (2009) quote an 1849 study of "insanity" in the Philadelphia penitentiary as identifying 16 percent of inmates in this category. Over 150 years later, Ditton (1999) reported 16 percent of offenders in state departments of correction had a mental disorder. For US federal institutions, Magaletta *et al.* (2009) reported that 15.2 percent of newly committed offenders at all levels of security and regions of the country had a mental illness. Their definition was based on a combination of a history of inpatient psychiatric care, psychotropic medication use and diagnosis of a serious mental illness. Data were based on intake forms and psychological intake screening. Female offenders had, on average, twice the rate of serious mental illness compared to males. This difference was considerably reduced if antidepressant medication use was excluded from the psychotropic medication use variable. The fact that one in seven male offenders (or one in four female offenders) may require mental health services suggests, Magaletta *et al.* indicate, that female and medium- and high-security facilities should be especially considered for such services. Given these data and their relative stability over time, it is apparent that any correctional system must provide adequately trained staff to screen, assess, manage, treat and organize services and programs to meet their needs (Magaletta *et al.*, 2009).

Requests for psychological services in prisons

Requests for psychological services on admission to prison follow a different pattern from the epidemiology of mental illness. Diamond *et al.* (2008) in the southern United States looked at over 2,600 male and female prisoners and found that one-tenth requested psychological services on admission. They note that a combination of prior mental health treatment and current symptoms are the most prominent factors associated with such a request. Specifically, males with a history of head injury who had previous mental health treatment, and those with symptoms of depression, hopelessness, nervousness, sleeping problems and racing thoughts were most likely to request treatment. Diamond *et al.*'s (2008) data indicate that the most commonly reported symptoms among male requesters were sleep problems (63 percent), nervousness (57 percent), depression (55 percent) and racing thoughts (35 percent). For female requesters, the most commonly reported symptoms were sleep problems (81 percent), depression (76 percent), nervousness (73 percent) and headaches (52 percent). It is apparent that this combination of previous susceptibility and a poor psychological reaction to imprisonment are good predictors of requesting treatment, along with demographic factors such as better education and older age, and with more positive help-seeking attitudes (Skogstad *et al.*, 2006). Diamond *et al.* (2008) also reported that African Americans in their US sample were 1.5 times more likely to request psychological services than all other races.

From a public health perspective, Diamond *et al.* argue that the correctional context provides an ideal opportunity to address the mental health needs of a high-need population that is often under-served or hard to reach in the community. They also suggest that the availability and accessibility of mental health care in the correctional context may exceed that in the communities from which the offenders come, and where insurance requirements, fees for service, and transportation issues may act as barriers. That is, the prison actually serves as a remediation for lack of community services and barriers to access. This is almost exactly parallel to the situation for physical health issues.

Traumatic brain injury in prisons

Previous head injuries are common among offenders, and in some samples more than 80 percent of inmates report at least one, and over half report multiple head injuries (Diamond *et al.*, 2007). The high prevalence of head injury or traumatic brain injury (TBI) suggests that it is important to assess frequency and severity of head injury and the level of impairment and disability arising from it. Such impairment may include psychological and behavioral difficulties, including those associated with criminal behavior. Diamond *et al.* developed a brief questionnaire on levels of head injury and outcomes of head injury in US offender populations, and found their TBIQ (Traumatic Brain Injury Questionnaire) to be a reliable and valid measure of frequency and severity of symptoms and of cognitive, psychological and behavioral functioning associated with TBI. It is important to be aware of the potential for TBI in offender populations and, if possible, to screen for it on admission or shortly thereafter.

Substance abuse treatment

There is a close correspondence between substance abuse, crime and incarceration. Indeed, drug treatment cuts crime rates more effectively than prison (Jones, 1999). Reporting on a British study, Jones indicates that monitoring 1,100 people who entered drug treatment programs (mainly heroin users) showed that they had committed about 70,000 crimes in the three months before treatment. Two years later, incidence of both drugs and criminal behavior was reduced by about half. Similar results in the United States suggest that for every dollar spent on drug misuse treatment, three dollars associated with the cost of crime were saved. Jones goes on to note that one-third of all thefts, burglaries and street robberies in England and Wales are drug-related. It is apparent that the solution should ideally lie in community treatment – for example, in the successful drug courts established in many jurisdictions in the United States.

Given these data, it could be concluded that prison is not the place for drug treatment. However, for subsequent offenses, the option of community treatment is not available and incarceration is often mandatory. Appropriately funded and staffed, drug treatment in prison may be an important option, perhaps with the advantage that the drug users are more likely to be sober and focused in prison. In a US study in the federal prison system, Magaletta *et al.* (2010) report that the criminal justice system makes nearly half of the referrals to community-based substance abuse treatment. They also note that substance abuse is frequently a chronic relapsing condition requiring repeated treatment episodes, and cyclical in its nature. In their sample, the frequency of pre-incarceration drug abuse treatment was similar for men and women, 31 percent and 35 percent, respectively. The figures for any prior drug treatment or program participation were 56 percent for state offenders and 46 percent for federal offenders. However, they also suggest that serious questions remain about the quality, ability and sustainability of the community-based treatment infrastructure, and that receipt of "treatment" and its nature may have been quite variable. Given their argument that the average drug career lasts 27 years and the average substance abuse treatment career lasts nine years, there is a need for repeated and sustained care including during incarceration.

Treatment capacity in US state prisons is quite inadequate relative to need, and about one-third of male and half of female prisoners will need residential treatment (Belenko and Peugh, 2005). There is, however, a wide variation in the mode and delivery of drug abuse treatment to incarcerated populations, and it is estimated that between 66 percent and 78 percent of *untreated* prisoners with heroin addiction histories relapse (Nurco *et al.*, 1991). In a randomized-assignment clinical trial of treatments in recently released prisoners in the United States, Kinlock *et al.* (2007) found very significant differences in three groups of prisoners, recruited between three and six months before release. The relapse rates (urine positive for opioids one month after release) for counseling only were 63 percent; for counseling plus transfer to a methadone-maintenance program on release from prison, 41 percent; and for counseling plus methadone maintenance started in prison, 28 percent. These data are telling: counseling alone (12 weekly sessions) was significantly worse (both statistically and clinically) in its outcome than starting methadone maintenance on release, and there was a very high success rate with methadone maintenance that was commenced a few months before release. It is clear that in terms of effectiveness, drug substitution (and particularly methadone for heroin users) has a major effect on reducing both heroin re-addiction and criminal behavior (since criminal behavior is closely tied to drug abuse and the need to obtain money for drugs). In a subsequent study, Gordon *et al.* (2008) found that this effect was maintained at six months. This approach will be the approach of choice in jurisdictions where methadone substitution therapy is possible, but not so where inmates and drug treatment professionals are limited in their treatment options by the philosophical views of politicians and administrators on drug substitution therapy. Nevertheless, therapeutic communities and counseling approaches are still 1.4 and 1.5 times more likely to reduce re-offending (Chandler *et al.*, 2009). Volunteer-led self-help organizations such as

Alcoholics Anonymous and Narcotics Anonymous are also effective in supporting recovery efforts at minimal cost.

It is also important to realize that drug treatment needs to be tailored to the needs of the inmate. Simpson and McNulty (2008) note that the needs of women drug users are very different to those of men, with women having more social problems which are amplified by higher stigma. Such concerns include pregnant women being reluctant to access antenatal services because of judgmental or hostile reaction of treatment professionals, and for drug-using mothers the fear of having children removed from their care.

Motivation is also crucial in successful treatment. Community-based studies have indicated that both engagement in treatment and retention in treatment are strongly predicted by motivation for treatment. A person who is not "ready for treatment" is unlikely to benefit. Hiller *et al.* (2009) note that this relationship between treatment and motivation is as relevant in incarcerated populations in the community. They report that greater problem severity (including incarceration) was associated with higher motivation for treatment scores in prison populations, suggesting that people with more drug-related life problems (including imprisonment) are more likely to recognize the need for help in beginning long-term recovery.

On the other hand, treatment in criminal justice settings is very different from that in free-world community settings in a number of ways. McCarty and Chandler (2009) review the evidence for organizational factors impacting treatment in prisons and note that while drug *education* services are common in US prisons and jails, more intensive treatment services are present in a minority of institutions (29 percent of prisons and 27 percent of jails offer therapeutic communities and only 11 percent of prisons and 1 percent of jails offer more than 26 hours per week of group counseling). State prisons tend to offer more intensive services, and facilities are more likely to use evidence-based practices when administrators see value and benefit in addiction and treatment services. It is debatable whether detoxification on its own can be considered "treatment," although it is a crucial clinical service that needs to be offered. It seems, McCarty and Chandler point out, that criminal justice entities have lower requirements for staff qualifications in the treatment area, and that as a consequence offenders may be getting a lower quality of care. The requirement, they argue, is to have interventions that integrate community, prison or jail, and probation and parole services so that treatment is as seamless as possible, and that a central focus (especially on re-integration into the community) should be on treatment as well as on criminal justice requirements. In some countries, such as the UK, there has been considerable emphasis on joining up drug treatment and criminal justice system interventions, and this model appears to be a productive one (Simpson and McNulty, 2008).

There is a growing recognition that addictions involve long-lasting and clear changes in brain circuitry that makes addicts very vulnerable to relapse, and that they are not simply a psychological condition but a brain disorder, with a significant genetic component (Chandler *et al.*, 2009). Increasingly, treatment interventions will also require an integration of the medical with the psychological to achieve maximum efficacy. One must also consider the collision between a primarily penal perspective on addicts and their crimes, as opposed to a perception of them as a primarily mental health concern. This collision may be played out as a conflict between treatment staff and custodial or administrative staff, particularly where they are employed by different organizations with different philosophies.

At a policy level, these organizational (and essentially cultural) issues can be approached by provision of more and better-trained staff. A plan which takes promising correctional staff and provides them with scholarship or educational opportunities to be trained in psychology or addiction treatment service provision is one way of meeting this need. In addition to bridging the cultural gap between criminal justice and treatment services, this also provides career enhancement opportunities for correctional staff, who often have a better understanding of prison culture and organization than outside staff.

At a public health level, addiction treatment in jails and prisons is unquestionably important. Apart from the individual benefit of treatment in reducing distress, there are clear benefits in vastly reduced crime, including violent crime where the victims are members of the community, and in health outcomes. These health outcomes include reduced risk of HIV and Hepatitis B and C infections and other blood-borne diseases, injection-site abscesses, where substance abusers are injecting unsafely, and the psychological costs to the families and friends of drug abusers. Within prisons, inmates who continue to obtain drugs are likely to inject unsafely and, as with outside drug abuse, are vulnerable to morbidity and mortality from adulterated, impure or over-pure drugs.

Improving public health and safety involves effectively treating drug abuse and addiction in the criminal justice system (Chandler *et al.*, 2009). However, most prisoners who could benefit from drug abuse treatment do not receive it. As Chandler *et al.* note, "Punishment alone is a futile and ineffective response to drug abuse, failing as a public safety intervention for offenders whose criminal behavior is directly related to drug use." There is a wealth of data on evidence-based treatment for drug offenders in criminal justice populations (Fletcher and Chandler, 2006) and it is consistent in establishing the effectiveness of such treatment in reducing threats to public and personal health in inmates. The challenge in many jurisdictions remains more one of political and organizational indifference or hostility and associated lack of funding than one of scientific evidence and the difficulties of implementing treatment in a correctional setting. There are increasing efforts to integrate drug treatment and criminal justice systems in countries such as the UK and in western Europe, and these point the way to a number of demonstration projects and best-practice models for correctional settings.

Incarcerogenic mental health

Mental health in prisons can be divided into three categories: that which is brought into the prison by the inmate; that which is latent in the inmate but is triggered or exacerbated by the prison situation; and that which is newly created by the prison. The latter two categories I call "incarcerogenic" mental health (that is, caused by the prison or imprisonment). This can in turn be divided into that which dissipates when the inmate is released; and that which leaves a permanent mental health problem. Liebling *et al.* (2005), talking about prison suicide risk, use the classification of imported risk (bringing the elevated suicide risk into prison with them), deprivation (caused by prison-induced distress) and a combined model (exposing vulnerable people to additional risk), which is a similar model in terms of the origin of the problem.

King (2005) provides an extreme but informative look at the effects of prison environment on mental health. In his description of the effects of supermax custody, he notes that there may be responses to sensory deprivation, including hypersensitivity to noise and other external stimuli, affective disturbances including shortness of breath, tachycardia and headaches, difficulties with thinking, concentration and memory, disturbances of thought, and problems with impulse control. Where prisoners were taken out for 24 hours, symptoms rapidly diminished (and presumably return with a return to solitary confinement). The effects of sensory deprivation appear to occur in any confinement lasting longer than ten days; King quotes Haney and Lynch (1997) as listing the following effects of increases in negative attitudes and affect: insomnia, anxiety, panic, withdrawal, hypersensitivity, ruminations, cognitive dysfunction, hallucinations, loss of control, aggression, rage, paranoia, hopelessness, lethargy, depression, emotional breakdowns, self-mutilation and suicidal impulses. Clearly, conditions that amount to sensory deprivation are unacceptable. On the other hand, King (2005) also notes that supermax that does not have sensory deprivation did, for some prisoners, provide some positive aspects, including giving people time to think and reflect, learn patience and control and give an opportunity to make decisions away from the influence of peers. At the other extreme, about one-fifth of inmates interviewed believed that the supermax experience had made them much worse and that they would come out more bitter and vengeful.

It is also crucial, King (2005) notes, that we consider the impact of prison environment on prison staff, and here he makes some interesting observations. In English close-supervision centers (the supermax equivalent), staff found their job stressful. In US supermax facilities, staff found their jobs less stressful than in other prisons (and often boring). He speculates that this is because staff in supermax settings in the United States have little to disturb their equilibrium.

Haney (2001) has described the psychological impact of incarceration with particular attention to their longer-term implications for post-prison adjustment. He found that dependence on the institution (institutionalization or prisonization) develops and that ex-inmates have compromised ability to do things on their own. Hypervigilance, distrust and suspicion also develop as a protection against people taking advantage of their weakness, and shaping a tough outer image requires emotional over-control, with alienation and social distancing adaptive in prison (the so-called "prison mask") but maladaptive on release. Haney also notes social withdrawal and isolation, and flatness of response, reminiscent of clinical depression. Incorporation of the exploitive norms of prison culture may include hypermasculinity and glorification of force and domination, which can be difficult to relinquish on release. Finally, diminished sense of self-worth and personal value arise from internalization of the prison experience, leading to a post-traumatic stress reaction to the pains of imprisonment in some prisoners. It is clear that the incarcerogenic mental health dysfunctions that may be generated in prisons may remain long after release.

Mental health in prisons is closely based on environmental factors, including staff–inmate interaction. Nurse *et al.* (2003) report that the primary negative impact on mental health was the impact of isolation and lack of activity – nothing to do, no mental stimulation and little opportunity to engage in education or skills/job training in some facilities. This led to extreme stress, anger and frustration. In such contexts, drug misuse in prison was one of the only options to "cope" as a mental escape. In many cases, lack of family contact or ability to maintain contact was also a source of anxiety. However, social contacts in prisons – both other inmates and staff – were a major source of incarcerogenic mental distress. Bullying by other prisoners and by staff were a major (and largely preventable) source of poor mental health generated inside the institution. As Nurse *et al.* (2003) point out, this leads to a cycle of stress, since inmates will often make things difficult for non-responsive or abusive officers, leading to staff stress, absenteeism and short-staffing, which places an additional burden on the remaining staff, and less time to deal with prisoners. This contribution to poor inmate mental health by staff is also emphasized by Liebling *et al.* (2005) with regard to prison suicide.

Mention should also be made of so-called "biochemical repression," where inmates are kept tranquilized by use or over-use of psychotropic medications. While this may be necessary on a temporary basis, it is inadvisable for long periods, and if it is used for long periods, it is a sure sign that something is amiss in the prison. There should be opportunities for inmates to occupy themselves – whether work, watching television or other activities – without having to resort to pharmacological shackles.

Suicide in prisoners

Suicide (and attempted suicide) rates are elevated well above population levels in prisoners in most western countries. Fazel *et al.* (2008) report that the rate is elevated some eight times in the United States, and (age-standardized) in England and Wales five times higher and increasing. Further, these rates remain after release – three- to four-fold higher in released prisoners compared to the general population in one US study. In a meta-analysis of 34 studies, Fazel *et al.* found that a combination of demographic, criminological and clinical factors predicted suicides. The odds ratios (the increased odds that a factor provides for suicide, the higher the odds ratio the more important the factor; no increased odds is 1.0, 2.0 doubles the risk, and so on) for suicide for each factor were: history of suicidal ideation, 15.2; history of attempted suicide, 8.4; having a current psychiatric diagnosis, 5.9; receiving psychotropic medication, 4.2; and having a history of alcohol use problems, 3.0.

Completed suicides in the California Department of Corrections over a six-year period were reviewed by Patterson and Hughes (2008). They found that prisoners who committed suicide were similar in age distribution and mental health factors to those who commit suicide in the community. However, other issues relating to incarceration, including single-cell accommodation, isolation and punitive sanctions, severely restricted living conditions and conditions of deprivation, or imposition of new charges or unexpected sentences, were also associated with suicide. They concluded that 60 percent of all prison suicides in this period were foreseeable (presence of elevated or high risk) or preventable. Caucasian prisoners and those with histories of suicide attempts, with safety concerns and anxiety or agitation, severe personality disorder and co-existing mental illness, are all at elevated risk.

In adolescents, however, predictors may be somewhat different. Hayes (2009) summarized a US national study on juvenile suicide in confinement, and found that they were evenly distributed in time, not just in the first few days of confinement, and most occurred in traditional waking hours, by hanging. Only 17 percent were on suicide watch. There was a strong association between room confinement and suicide, but none with intoxication with drugs or alcohol. However, suicide prevention resources were notably lacking in juvenile detention centers.

There is a clear interaction between distress (in its extreme form leading to suicide attempts or completed suicides) and staff–inmate interactions. Such interactions may in a negative form trigger or create distress, or in a positive form prevent or reduce distress. Liebling *et al.* (2005) argue that a significant contribution to prisoner distress and suicide is made by "uneven experiences of unfairness, disrespect and lack of safety" (p. 209). Their argument that suicide is caused by prison-induced distress is based on a legitimacy-related argument. Legitimacy encompasses considerations of fairness and respect and is central to perceptions of impartiality of punishment. Where the inmate sees the behavior of the prison staff as unfair (King [2005] notes that most prisoners have a profound sense of justice and fair play), then they also see themselves as not receiving justice, but arbitrary punitive attacks or gratuitous harassment. Liebling *et al.* propose that levels of distress and rates of suicide in prisons are related to levels of respect and fairness, and safety and predictability, in particular prisons.

As part of their study of moral performance in prisons, Liebling *et al.* measured levels of distress in 12 prisons in England and Wales. The highest levels of distress were found in those with imported vulnerability, women, unsentenced prisoners, black and Asian prisoners, and those who were in that prison for the first time. They note that there is an interaction between vulnerable persons and high-risk situations (person–prison interaction). There were high levels of distress in the first month, which declined over time. Taking each prison by year, they found very high correlations (around 0.80) between individual-level distress and prison-level suicide rates. The measures that contributed most to overall distress were perceived physical safety, respect, relationships with and fairness of prison staff, dignity, frustration, clarity, security and order and family contact. Perceived safety had both a direct and a mediating role given that a prison is a high-threat, low-control environment. As Liebling *et al.* note, it is necessary to consider how and whether inmate psychological and physical well-being might be accomplished in the prison, and if not, why not.

Prevention of suicide in prison and suicide prevention programs in prisons is a sentinel index of the adequacy of mental health services. Daniel (2006) notes that suicide prevention is a collaborative responsibility of administrative, custodial and clinical staff and must incorporate identification of risk, assessment, evaluation, treatment, preventive intervention and training of all medical, mental health and custodial staff. Suicide risk rating scores should be available on all inmates after arrival and placed in medical and custodial records. A "watch-take" policy for administration of psychotropic medications is necessary, and administrative management including segregation monitoring, offender assignment and cell design should be included. Monitoring of inter-facility movement is also necessary as temporary placements may be used to less-supervised settings like courts.

Suicide prevention training packages such as the STORM program (Skills-based Training On Risk Management) is one package developed for England and Wales which emphasizes practice and review of interactions with potentially suicidal prisoners (Hayes *et al.*, 2008). The two days training of trainers was evaluated using the Attitude to Suicide Prevention Scale (Herron and Ticehurst, 2001) and significant increases in attitudes, knowledge and confidence relating to suicide prevention were found after the course and maintained after 6–8 months. However, Hayes *et al.* also recommend refresher training after 12–18 months.

Public health and mental health in prisons

Mental health in correctional settings has a number of public health dimensions. First, it provides an opportunity for screening and treatment of serious mental illness that may not have been identified in the community. Second, personality disorders and other Axis-II problems are common in correctional facilities. Among the conditions identified in correctional settings is TBI, which is frequently occurring but very rarely screened for in correctional settings, and may have major implications for criminal behavior or managing tasks of daily living. Thus, correctional facilities have a major role in screening and treating mental illness and brain injury.

Given the high number of drug users in prison and jail, treatment for drug and alcohol addiction should be a significant focus of such facilities, particularly given the close relationship between addiction and crime. Effective drug and alcohol treatment programs in correctional facilities which are closely linked to continuation of treatment on return to the community are the most likely to work.

Perhaps the clearest aspect of mental health in prisons is that associated with suicide or attempted suicide in prisons. The health promotion aspect of suicide in prisons is most closely associated with education of correctional staff to carry out risk assessment and monitoring of inmates at risk of suicide. The second crucial aspect of health promotion activities in prisons is the need for prison staff to understand the incarcerogenic dimension of mental health and how unfair and arbitrary actions and bullying on the part of prison staff or other inmates has a lasting and very negative impact on mental health of inmates. In addition to this, unfair and arbitrary behavior on the part of prison staff simply de-legitimizes the correctional experience in the eyes of the inmate. Thus, for mental health aspects of incarceration, the health promotion interventions may need to be targeted at correctional staff more than at inmates.

10 Conclusions

Some principles of public health and health in prisons

In this book, I have tried to sketch out the issues, from the perspectives of health and medicine, occupational health and safety, law, management, criminology, sociology, human rights, and history, which underlie health and public health in correctional settings. Simply, these include the following:

1 For infectious diseases and mental health issues, prisons can form an incubator for transmission of pathogens and exacerbation of poor health.
2 Prisoners are part of the community from which they come into prison to which the vast majority will return. They bring in pre-existing health problems and frequently take new ones back to their community.
3 Staff and inmates form part of the same prison environment and community from a health and disease point of view. Dealing with the health of one group and not the other is an artificial distinction when both are part of the same correctional community. Health problems are taken back to the community and family by both inmates and staff.
4 The physical environment of the prison can contain many occupational and safety problems for both staff and for inmates. Many of these can be remedied by physical change in the fabric, or organizational practices in the correctional environment.
5 Most inmates come from the most disadvantaged sector of the community and will concentrate physical health and mental health disadvantages. Many will have missed out on basic health care and health education and have remediable health problems.
6 Peer education for inmates is perhaps the best opportunity we have to extend health knowledge and awareness not only within the correctional setting, but also to their family and contacts in the free world who are equally likely to come from disadvantaged settings.
7 Health education and remedial care can constitute a form of restorative justice at a population as well as an individual level by returning inmates to the community healthier and with lowered health risk behaviours.
8 People are sent to prison as punishment, not for punishment: they are not sentenced to poor health care and inadequate medical treatment and

it forms no part of their punishment. Approaches to health and health care of inmates are, however, usually highly influenced by the health system context and ideology of the state where they are incarcerated.

9 The body can and sometimes does become a locus for punitive health care, lack of treatment, or torture. Such conduct violates inmates' status as humans and indeed also brings into question the humanity of those who violate the ethical standards of care.

10 Mental health issues in prison settings are as important as physical and environmental health ones. Mental health problems can be both brought in from the free world, and created in correctional settings. There is significant overlap between crime and mental illness and sometimes prisons will have disproportionately large populations with mental health issues, and serve as mental hospitals of last resort.

11 Prisons are by definition a health setting, either for good or for bad. Healthy or healthier prisons are attainable even in resource-poor settings and there is probably no prison, even in the absence of funding, where significant improvement in the health and safety of staff and inmates is not possible.

12 Public health in prisons requires buy-in at managerial, staff, health care worker, and inmate levels and often at a political level as well. Correctional settings are a system where, despite appearances and regimented regimes, health improvement and health care are difficult to impose and easy to sabotage. They need to be seen to be above punitive health philosophies in the interests of all, including management, community, staff and inmates.

Public health and health care are an integral part of correctional practice and indeed criminology, and should be recognized as part of health rehabilitation, planning and management. While not all people will agree with all of these principles, they to a greater or lesser extent can guide better health for all, at individual and community levels, in jails, prisons and other correctional settings.

Notes

Chapter 4

1 Page numbers refer to the Westlaw © summary of *Ruiz* v. *Estelle*, 131 pages, where the first 21 pages are headnotes. The case conclusion commences at 1274 Introduction, p. 22

Chapter 5

1 The "denial of medical care may result in pain and suffering which no one suggests would serve any penological purpose … the infliction of such unnecessary suffering is inconsistent with contemporary standards of decency" (*Estelle* v. *Gamble* [429 U.S. at 103, 97 S.Ct. at 290]).

Chapter 6

1 A version of this chapter was published in the *Journal of Correctional Health*, 2011, 17:6–18. Reproduced with kind permission.
2 We sat with a group of 28 inmates in a prison classroom equipped with a whiteboard and markers and asked them to generate health topics that they would like to know more about, and which were personally important to them. They are listed in the order generated.

Chapter 7

1 A version of this chapter was published in the *Prison Service Journal*, 2010, 192:55–59. Reproduced with kind permission.

Chapter 8

1 A version of this chapter was published in the *International Journal of Prisoner Health*, 2012, 8:16–27. Reproduced with kind permission.

References

Alarid LF (2009). Risk factors for potential occupational exposure to HIV: A study of correctional officers. *Journal of Criminal Justice*, 37:114–122.

Alvarez-Dardet C, Montahud C, Ruiz MT (2001). The widening social class gap of preventive health behaviors in Spain. *European Journal of Public Health*, 11:225–226.

Armstrong GS, Griffin ML (2004). Does the job matter? Comparing correlates of stress among treatment and correctional staff in prisons. *Journal of Criminal Justice*, 32:577–592.

Baillargeon J, Wu H, Kelley M, Grady J, Linthicum L, Dunn K (2003). Hepatitis C seroprevalence among newly incarcerated inmates in the Texas correctional system. *Public Health* 117:43–48.

Baillargeon J, Binswanger IA, Penn JV, Williams BA, Murray OJ (2009a). Psychiatric disorders and repeat incarcerations: The revolving prison door. *American Journal of Psychiatry*, 166(1):103–109.

Baillargeon J, Penn JV, Thomas CR, Temple JR, Baillargeon G, Murray OJ (2009b). Psychiatric disorders and suicide in the nation's largest state prison system. *Journal of the American Academy of Psychiatry and the Law*, 37(2):188–193.

Baillargeon J, Penn JV, Knight K, Harzke AJ, Baillargeon G, Becker EA (2010). Risk of reincarceration among prisoners with co-occurring severe mental illness and substance use disorders. *Administration and Policy in Mental Health*, 37(4):367–374.

Balz D (1981, November 7). US seeks delay in civil rights lawsuit against Texas prisons. *Washington Post*, p. A5.

Bandura A (1986). *Social Foundations of Thought and Action: A Social Cognitive Theory*. Englewood Cliffs, NJ: Prentice-Hall.

Belenko S, Peugh J (2005). Estimating drug treatment needs among state prison inmates. *Drug and Alcohol Dependence*, 77:269–281.

Bentham J (1789 [1996]). Introduction to the principles of morals and legislation. In: Burns JH, Hart HLA (eds.) *The Collected Works of Jeremy Bentham*. Oxford: Oxford University Press, p. 283.

Binswanger IA, White MC, Pérez-Stable EJ, Goldenson J, Tulsky JP (2005). Cancer screening among jail inmates: Frequency, knowledge and willingness. *American Journal of Public Health*, 95:1781–1787.

Binswanger IA, Stern MF, Deyo RA, Heagerty PJ, Cheadle A, Elmore JG, Koespell TD (2007). Release from prison: A high risk of death for former inmates. *New England Journal of Medicine*, 356:157–165.

Binswanger IA, Krueger PM, Steiner JF (2009). Prevalence of chronic medical conditions among jail and prison inmates in the USA compared with the general population. *Journal of Epidemiology and Community Health*, 63:912–919.

Brown M (2009). *The Culture of Punishment: Prison, Society and Spectacle*. New York: New York University Press.

Burns T (1992). *Erving Goffman*. London: Routledge.

Butler S (1872 [1934]). *Erewhon*. Norwalk, CT: Easton Press.

Byers B (1982, May 16). Wrong way to handle prison crisis. *Houston Post*, p. 3.

Carroll L (1999). *Lawful Order: A Case History of Correctional Crisis and Reform*. New York: Garland.

Chandler RK, Fletcher BW, Volkow ND (2009). Treating drug abuse and addiction in the criminal justice system: Improving public health and safety. *Journal of the American Medical Association*, 301(2):183–190.

Cheliotis LK (2012). Suffering at the hands of the state: Conditions of imprisonment and prisoner health in contemporary Greece. *European Journal of Criminology*, 9:3–22.

Clapham A (2007). *Human Rights: A Very Short Introduction*. Oxford: Oxford University Press.

Collins M (1988). Prison education: A substantial metaphor for adult education practice. *Adult Education Quarterly*, 38:101–110.

Commission for Healthcare Audit and Inspection and HM Inspectorate of Prisons (2009). *Commissioning Healthcare in Prisons*. London: Healthcare Commission.

Coninx R, Maher D, Reyes H, Grzemska M (2000). Tuberculosis in prisons in countries with high prevalence. *British Medical Journal*, 320:440–442.

Conklin TJ, Lincoln T, Flanigan TP (1998). A public health model to connect correctional health care with communities. *American Journal of Public Health* 88:1249–1250.

Crawford DH (2007). *Deadly Companions: How Microbes Shaped our History*. Oxford: Oxford University Press.

Daniel AE (2006). Preventing suicide in prison: a collaborative responsibility of administrative, custodial, and clinical staff. *Journal of the American Academy of Psychiatry and Law*, 34:165–175.

Darlington I (1955). Southwark prisons. *Survey of London: Volume 25: St George's Fields (The Parishes of St. George the Martyr Southwark and St. Mary Newington)*, pp. 9–21. From British History Online: www.british-history.ac.uk (accessed 2011).

Department of Health (2006). *Clinical Management of Drug Dependence in the Adult Prison Setting*. London: HM Stationery Office.

Diamond PM, Harzke AJ, Magaletta PR, Cummins AG, Frankowski R (2007). Screening for traumatic brain injury in an offender sample: A first look at the reliability and validity of the Traumatic Brain Injury Questionnaire. *Journal of Head Trauma and Rehabilitation*, 22:330–338.

Diamond PM, Magaletta PR, Harzke AJ, Baxter J (2008). Who requests psychological services upon admission to prison? *Psychological Services*, 5:97–107.

Ditton PM (1999). *Mental Health and Treatment of Offenders and Probationers*. Washington, DC: Bureau of Justice Statistics Bulletin, US Department of Justice.

Dolan K, Hall W, Wodak A (1996). Methadone maintenance reduces injecting in prison. *British Medical Journal*, 312:1162.

Dolan K, Lowe D, Shearer J (2004). Evaluation of the condom distribution program in New South Wales prisons, Australia. *Journal of Law, Medicine & Ethics*, 32:124–128.

Duff A (2003). Restoration and retribution. In: von Hirsch A, Roberts J, Bottoms A, Roach K, Schiff M (eds.), *Restorative Justice and Criminal Justice: Competing or Reconcilable Paradigms?* Oxford: Hart Publishing, pp. 43–59.

Elliott R (2007). Deadly disregard: Government refusal to implement evidence-based measures to prevent HIV and Hepatitis C virus infections in prisons. *Canadian Medical Association Journal*, 177:262–264.

Ellis DG, Mayrose J, Phelan M (2006). Consultation times in emergency telemedicine using realtime videoconferencing. *Journal of Telemedicine and Telecare*, 12:303–305.

Fazel S, Danesh J (2002). Serious mental disorder in 23,000 prisoners: A systematic review of 62 surveys. *The Lancet*, 359(9306):545.

Fazel S, Cartwright J, Norman-Nott A, Hawton K (2008). Suicide in prisoners: A systematic review of the literature. *Journal of Clinical Psychiatry*, 69:1721–1731.

Fisher JE, O'Donohue WT (eds.) (2006). *Practitioner's Guide to Evidence-Based Psychotherapy*. New York: Springer.

Fletcher BW, Chandler RK (2006). *Principles of Drug Abuse Treatment for Criminal Justice Populations*. Washington, DC: National Institute on Drug Abuse.

Foucault M (1977). *Discipline and Punish: The Birth of the Prison*. (A. Sheridan trans.). New York: Vintage.

Franks Z (1981, January 18). Justice: devil-saint Federal Judge. *Houston Chronicle*, pp. 1, 14.

Freire P (1972). *Pedagogy of the Oppressed* (MB Ramos, trans.). Harmondsworth: Penguin.

Freire P, Macedo D (1993). *Pedagogy of the City*. New York: Continuum.

Gadotti M (1994). *Reading Paulo Freire: His Life and Work* (J Milton, trans.). Albany, NY: SUNY Press.

Garland D (1990). *Punishment and Modern Society*. Oxford: Clarendon Press.

Gilbert M (1991). *Churchill: A Life*. London: Heinemann.

Goffman E (1956). *The Presentation of Self in Everyday Life*. New York: Doubleday.

Goffman E (1961). *Asylums*. New York: Anchor.

Gordon MS, Kinlock TW, Schwartz RP, O'Grady KE (2008). A randomized trial of methadone maintenance for prisoners: Findings at 6 months post-release. *Addiction*, 103:1333–1342.

Greenberg E, Dunleavy E, Kutner M, White S (2007). *Literacy Behind Bars: Results from the 2003 National Association of Adult Literacy Prison Survey (NCES 2007–473)*. Washington, DC: National Center for Educational Statistics.

Greifinger R (ed.) (2010). *Public Health Behind Bars: From Prisons to Communities*. New York: Springer.

Haney C (2001). The psychological impact of incarceration: Implications for post-prison adjustment. Online. Available at: http://aspe.hhs.gov/hsp/prison2home02/haney.htm (accessed February 11, 2012).

Haney C (2005). The contextual revolution in psychology and the question of prison effects. In: Liebling A, Maruna S (eds.), *The Effects of Imprisonment*. Cullompton: Willan, pp. 66–93.

Hardy A (1995). Development of the prison medical service, 1774–1895. In: Creese R, Bynum WF, Bearn J (eds.), *The Health of Prisoners: Historical Essays*. Amsterdam: Rodopi, pp. 59–80.

Harpham T, Burton S, Blue I (2001). Healthy city projects in developing countries: The first evaluation. *Health Promotion International*, 16:111–125.

Hart CL, Davey Smith G, Blane D (1998). Inequalities in mortality by social class measured at 3 stages of the lifecourse. *American Journal of Public Health*, 88:471–474.

Hart JT (1971). The inverse care law. *Lancet*, 1:405–412.

Harvard Law Review (2010). Constitutional law – Eighth amendment – Eastern District of California holds that prisoner release is necessary to remedy unconstitutional California prison conditions. *Harvard Law Review*, 123:752–759.

Harzke AJ, Ross MW, Scott DP (2006). Predictors of post release healthcare utilization among HIV positive inmates: A pilot study. *AIDS Care*, 18:290–301.

Harzke AJ, Baillargeon J, Pruitt SL, Paar DP, Pulvino JS, Kelley MF (2010). Prevalence of chronic medical conditions among inmates in the Texas prison system. *Journal of Urban Health*, 87:486–503.

Hayes AJ, Shaw JJ, Lever-Green G, Parker D, Gask L (2008). Improvements to suicide prevention training for prison staff in England and Wales. *Suicide and Life-Threatening Behavior*, 38:708–713.

Hayes LM (2009). Juvenile suicide in confinement: Findings from the first national survey. *Suicide and Life-Threatening Behavior*, 39:353–363.

Herron J, Ticehurst H (2001). Attitudes toward suicide prevention in front-line health staff. *Suicide and Life-Threatening Behavior*, 31:342–347.

Hessl SM (2001). Police and corrections. *Occupational Medicine*, 16(1):39–49.

Hiller ML, Narevic E, Webster M, Rosen P, Staton M, Leukefeld C, Garrity TF, Kayo R (2009). Problem severity and motivation for treatment in incarcerated substance abusers. *Substance Use and Misuse*, 44:28–41.

Hirst J (1995). The Australian experience: The convict colony. In: Morris N, Rothman DJ (eds.), *The Oxford History of the Prison: The Practice of Punishment in Western Society*, pp. 263–295.

HMIP (Inspectorate of Prisons for England and Wales) (1996). *Patient or Prisoner? A New Strategy for Health Care in Prisons*. London: Home Office.

HMPS/NHS (1999). *The Future Organization of Prison Care: Report by the Joint Prison Service and National Health Service Executive Working Group*. London: Department of Health.

Hopper CB (1969). *Sex in Prison: The Mississippi Experiment with Conjugal Visiting*. Baton Rouge, FL: Louisiana State University Press.

Houston Chronicle (1982, 15 January). Texas wins appeal on prison reform. p. 1.

Houston Chronicle (2009, October 20). Editorial. p. B13. Online. Available at: http://www.chron.com/CDA/archives/archive.mpl?id=2009_4801648 (accessed February 27, 2010).

Howard J (1784 [1929]). *The State of the Prisons*. London: Dent.

Hunter G (1980, December 13). Inmates suit to cost many millions. *Houston Chronicle*, pp. 1, 6, 10.

Jetté M, Sidney K (1991). The benefits and challenges of a fitness and lifestyle enhancement program for correctional officers. *Canadian Journal of Public Health*, 82: 46–51.

Joint Prison Service and National Health Service Executive Working Group (1999). *The Future Organization of Prison Care*. London: Department of Health.

Jones J (1999). Drug treatment beats prison for cutting crime and addiction rates. *British Medical Journal*, 319: 470.

King RD (2005). The effects of supermax custody. In: Liebling A, Maruna S (eds.), *The Effects of Imprisonment*. Cullompton: Willan, pp. 118–145.

King RD, McDermott K (1995). *The State of Our Prisons*. Oxford: Clarendon Press.

Kinlock TW, Gordon MS, Schwartz RP, O'Grady K, Fitzgerald TT, Wilson M (2007). A randomized clinical trial of methadone maintenance for prisoners: Results at 1-month post-release. *Drug and Alcohol Dependence*, 91:220–227.

Kinlock TW, Gordon MS, Schwartz RP, O'Grady KE (2008). A study of methadone maintenance for male prisoners: 3-month postrelease outcomes. *Criminal Justice and Behavior*, 35:34–47.

Kuhn TS (1970) *The Structure of Scientific Revolutions*. 2nd ed. Chicago, IL: University of Chicago Press.

Kunst AE, Bos V, Lahelma E, *et al.* (2005). Trends in socioeconomic inequalities in self-assessed health in 10 European countries. *International Journal of Epidemiology*, 34:295–305.

Lerner M, Simmons CH (1966). Observer reaction to the "innocent victim": Compassion or rejection? *Journal of Personality and Social Psychology*, 4:203–210.

Liebling A, Arnold H (2004). *Prisons and their Moral Performance: A Study of Values, Quality and Prison Life*. Oxford: Oxford University Press.

Liebling A, Durie L, Stiles A, Tait S (2005). Revisiting prison suicide: The role of fairness and distress. In: Liebling A, Maruna S (eds.), *The Effects of Imprisonment*. Cullompton: Willan, pp. 209–231.

Lifton RJ (2000). *The Nazi Doctors: Medical Killing and the Psychology of Genocide*. New York: Basic Books.

Lindquist CA, Whitehead JT (1986). Burnout, job stress and job satisfaction among southern correctional officers: Perception and causal factors. *Journal of Offender Counseling, Services and Rehabilitation*, 10(4):5–26.

Lindsley W (2008). 60 Am Jur 2d penal and correctional institutions §99. *American Jurisprudence*.

Livingstone S, Owen T, Macdonald A (2008). *Prison Law*. 4th ed. Oxford: Oxford University Press.

Madhukar P, Kalantri S, Aggarwal AN, Menzies D, Blumberg HM (2006). Nosocomial tuberculosis in India. *Emerging Infectious Diseases*, 12:1311–1318.

Magaletta PR, Diamond PM, Faust E, Daggett DM, Camp SD (2009). Estimating the mental illness component of service need in corrections: Results from the Mental Health Prevalence Project. *Criminal Justice and Behavior*, 36:229–244.

Magaletta PR, Diamond PM, Weinmann BM, Burnell A, Leukefeld CG (2010). Preentry substance abuse services: The heterogeneity of offender experiences. *Crime and Delinquency*, DOI: 10.1177/0011128710362055.

Martin SS, Butzin CA, Saum CA, Inciardi JA (1999). Three-year outcomes of therapeutic community treatment for drug-involved offenders in Delaware: From prison to work release to aftercare. *The Prison Journal*, 79:294–320.

Martín-Baró, I. (1994) *Writings for a Liberation Psychology* (edited by Aron A, Corne S). Cambridge, MA: Harvard University Press.

Maruna S (2001). *Making Good: How Ex-Convicts Reform and Rebuild Their Lives*. Washington, DC: American Psychological Association Books.

McCarty D, Chandler RK (2009). Understanding the importance of organizational and system variables on addiction treatment services within criminal justice settings. *Drug and Alcohol Dependence*, 103:S91–S93.

McConville S (1995). The Victorian prison: England, 1865–1965. In: Morris N, Rothman DJ (eds.), *The Oxford History of the Prison: The Practice of Punishment in Western Society*, pp. 131–167.

Møller L, Stöver H, Jürgens R, Gatherer A, Nikogosian H (eds.) (2007) *Health in Prisons: A WHO Guide to the Essentials in Prison Health*. WHO: Copenhagen.

Mullen PD, Cummins AG, Velasquez MM, von Sternberg K, Carvajal R (2003). Jails as important but constrained venues for addressing women's health. *Family and Community Health*, 26:157–168.

Mullen R, Rowland J, Arbiter N, Yablonsky L, Fleishman B (2001). California's first prison therapeutic community: A 10-year review. *Offender Substance Abuse Report*, 1(2):17–32.

Mutter RC, Grimes RM, Labarthe D (1994). Evidence of intraprison spread of HIV infection. *Archives of Internal Medicine*, 154:793–795.

National Center on Addiction and Substance Abuse (CASA) at Columbia University (2010). *Behind Bars II: Substance Abuse and America's Prison Population*. New York: Columbia University.

National Institute of Justice (2008). *Strategies to Prevent Prison Rape by Changing the Correctional Culture*. Washington, DC: National Institute of Justice.

National Institute of Medicine (2004). *Insuring America's Health: Principles and Recommendations*. Washington, DC: National Academies Press.

NCCHC (National Commission on Correctional Health Care) (2008). *Standards for Mental Health Services in Correctional Facilities*. Chicago, IL: NCCHC.

Nurco DN, Hanlon TE, Kinlock TW (1991). Recent research on the relationship between illicit drug use and crime. *Behavioral Science and Law*, 9:221–242.

Nurse J, Woodcock P, Ormsby J (2003). Influence of environmental factors on mental health within prisons: Focus group study. *British Medical Journal*, 327:480–483.

Ogińska-Bulik N (2005). The role of personal and social resources in preventing adverse health outcomes in employees of uniformed professions. *International Journal of Occupational Medicine and Environmental Health*, 18:233–240.

Okie S (2007). Sex, drugs, prisons, and HIV. *New England Journal of Medicine*, 356:105–108.

Osemene NI, Essien EJ, Egbunike IG (2001). HIV/AIDS behind bars: An avenue for culturally sensitive interventions. *Journal of the National Medical Association*, 93:481–486.

Paine T (1791). *Rights of Man: Answer to Mr. Burke's Attack on the French Revolution*. London: JS Jordan.

Parker GF (2009). Impact of a mental health training course for correctional officers on a special housing unit. *Psychiatric Services*, 60:640–645.

Patterson RF, Hughes K (2008). Review of completed suicides in the California Department of Corrections and Rehabilitation, 1999 to 2004. *Psychiatric Services*, 59:676–682.

Perkinson R (2010). *Texas Tough: The Rise of America's Prison Empire*. New York: Picador.

Peters EM (1995). Prison before the prison: The ancient and medieval worlds. In: Morris N, Rothman DJ (eds.), *The Oxford History of the Prison: The Practice of Punishment in Western Society*, pp. 3–47.

Porter R (1995). Howard's beginning: Prisons, disease, hygiene. In: Creese R, Bynum WF, Bearn J (eds.), *The Health of Prisoners: Historical Essays*. Amsterdam: Rodopi, pp. 5–26.

Ramsbotham D (1996). *Patient or Prisoner?* London: Home Office.

Ramsbotham D (2003). *Prisongate: The Shocking State of Britain's Prisons and the Need for Visionary Change*. London: Free Press.

Reavis DJ (1985, May). How they ruined our prisons. *Texas Monthly*, 13:153–160.

Reynolds C (2002). The final chapters of Ruiz v. Estelle. *Corrections Today*, June 1, 1–4.

Risser JMH, Risser WL, Gefter LR, Brandstetter DM, Cromwell PF (2001). Implementation of a screening program for Chlamydial infection in incarcerated adolescents. *Sexually Transmitted Diseases*, 28:43–46.

Risser WL, Smith KC (2005). Tuberculosis in incarcerated youth in Texas. *Journal of the American Medical Association*, 293:2716–2717.

Rodríguez CM, Marques LF, Touze G (2002). HIV and injection drug use in Latin America. *AIDS*, 16(3):S34–S41.

Romero O (1988). *The Violence of Love*. (Brockman JR, trans.). Farmington PA: Plough Publishing.

Ross MW (2010). Prison staff occupational health and safety and its relationship with inmate health: A review. *Prison Services Journal*, 192:55–59.

Ross MW (2011). Pedagogy for prisoners: An approach to peer health education for inmates. *Journal of Correctional Health Care*, 17:6–18.

Ross MW, Ferreira-Pinto JB (2000). Toward a public health of situations: The re-contextualization of risk. *Cadernos de Saúde Pública*, 16(1):59–71.

Ross MW, Kelly A (2000). Interventions to reduce HIV transmission in homosexual men. In Peterson JL, DiClemente RJ (eds.), *Handbook of HIV Prevention*. New York: Plenum, pp. 201–216.

Ross MW, Harzke AJ, Scott DP, McCann K, Kelley M (2006). Outcomes of project Wall Talk: An HIV/AIDS peer education program implemented within the Texas State Prison system. *AIDS Education and Prevention*, 18:504–517.

Ross MW, Liebling A, Tait S (2011). Inmate healthcare measurement, satisfaction and access in prisons: The relationships of prison climate to health service in correctional environments. *Howard Journal of Criminology*, 50:262–274.

Ryan W (1976). *Blaming the Victim*. New York: Vintage.

Schmidt U (2006). *Justice at Nuremburg: Leo Alexander and the Nazi Doctors' Trial*. New York: Palgrave Macmillan.

Schmidt U (2007). *Karl Brandt: Medicine and Power in the Third Reich*. London: Hambledon Continuum.

Senior J, Shaw J (2007). Prison healthcare. In: Jewkes Y (ed.), *Handbook on Prisons*. Willan: Cullompton, pp. 377–398.

Sim J (1990). *Medical Power in Prisons: The Prison Medical Service in England 1774–1989*. Milton Keynes: Open University Press.

Sim J (1995). The prison medical service and the deviant 1895–1948. In: Creese R, Bynum WF, Bearn J (eds.), *The Health of Prisoners: Historical Essays*. Amsterdam: Rodopi, pp. 102–115.

Simpson M, McNulty J (2008). Different needs: Women's drug use and treatment in the UK. *International Journal of Drug Policy*, 19:169–175.

Skogstad P, Deane FP, Spicer J (2006). Barriers to helpseeking among New Zealand prison inmates. *Journal of Offender Rehabilitation*, 42:1–24.

Smith C (2000). "Healthy prisons": A contradiction in terms? *Howard Journal of Criminal Justice*, 39:339–353.

Sourcebook of Criminal Justice Statistics (2001). Online. Available at: http://www.albany.edu/sourcebook (accessed 2011).

Spierenburg P (1995). The body and the state: Early modern Europe. In: Morris N, Rothman DJ (eds.), *The Oxford History of the Prison: The Practice of Punishment in Western Society*, pp. 49–77.

Spitz V (2005). *Doctors from Hell: The Horrific Accounts of Nazi Experiments on Humans*. Boulder, CO: Sentient.

Standley AJ (1995). Medical treatment and prisoners' health in Stafford Gaol during the eighteenth century. In: Creese R, Bynum WF, Bearn J (eds.), *The Health of Prisoners: Historical Essays*. Amsterdam: Rodopi, pp. 27–43.

Taylor P (1993). *The Texts of Paulo Freire*. Buckingham: Open University Press.

Texas Department of Criminal Justice (2006). Fiscal year 2006 statistical report. Online. Available at: http://www.tdcj.state.tx.us/publications/executive/FY_2006_Statistical_Report.pdf (accessed December 23, 2006).

Townsend P, Phillimore P, Beattie A (1988). *Health and Deprivation: Inequality and the North*. London: Croom Helm.

Trow L (1980, December 14). Judge demands TDC to alleviate unconstitutional conditions: Court. *Huntsville Item*, p. 1.

Tucker W, Olofson M, Simring S, Goodman W, Bienefeld S (2006). A pilot study of inmate preferences for on-site, visiting consultant, and telemedicine psychiatric services. *CNS Spectrums*, 11:783–787.

Turner BS (1996). *The Body and Society*. 2nd ed. London: Sage.

US Department of Health and Human Services (2000). *Healthy People 2010: Understanding and Improving Health*. 2nd ed. Washington, DC: US Government Printing Office.

Vara R (1982, May 23). TDC must face up to questions crisis raised. *Houston Post*, p. 5.

Virchow R. (1941) Introductory article, *Die medizinische Reform*. In Henry Ernest Sigerist, *Medicine and Human Welfare*. New Haven, CT: Yale University Press.

Walsh E (2009). The emotional labor of nurses working in Her Majesty's Prison Service. *Journal of Forensic Nursing*, 5:143–152.

Watson S (1994). Applying Foucault: Some problems encountered in the application of Foucault's methods to the history of medicine in prisons. In: Jones C, Porter R (eds.), *Reassessing Foucault: Power, Medicine and the Body*. London: Routledge, pp. 132–151.

West F (1981, November 14). Clements hoping for "compromise" on prison reform. *Houston Post*, p. 1.

Wexler HK, De Leon G, Thomas G, Kressel D, Peters J (1999). The Amity Prison TC evaluation reincarceration outcomes. *Criminal Justice and Behavior*, 26:147–167.

WHO (n.d.). Healthy settings. Online. Available at: http://www.whi.int/healthy_settings/en (accessed 2011).

WHO (2003). Delaration, Moscow, 24th October: Prison health as part of public health. Online. Available at: http://www.who.it/document/hipp/moscow_declaration_eng04.pdf (accessed February 8, 2010).

WHO (2007). Effectiveness of interventions to manage HIV in prisons: Provision of condoms and other measures to decrease sexual transmission. Online. Available at: http://www.who.int/hiv/idu/Prisons_condoms.pdf (accessed 2011).

Wiener MJ (1995). The health of prisoners and the two faces of Benthamism. In: Creese R, Bynum WF, Bearn J (eds.), *The Health of Prisoners: Historical Essays*. Amsterdam: Rodopi, pp. 44–58.

Wilkinson RG (1996). *Unhealthy Societies: The Afflictions of Inequality*. London: Routledge.

Wilper AP, Woolhandler S, Boyd JW, Lasser KE, McCormick D, Bor DH, Himmelstein DU (2009). The health and health care of US prisoners: Results of a nationwide survey. *American Journal of Public Health*, 99:666–671.

Wolfe MI, Xu F, Patel P, O'Cain M, Schillinger JA, St Louis ME, Finelli L (2001). An outbreak of syphilis in Alabama prisons: Correctional health policy and communicable disease control. *American Journal of Public Health*, 91:1220–1225.

Yorke J, Hethcote H, Nold A (1978). Dynamics and control of the transmission of gonorrhea. *Sexually Transmitted Diseases*, 5:51–56.

Young J (2002). Crime and social exclusion. In: Maguire M, Morgan R, Reiner R (eds.), *The Oxford Handbook of Criminology*. 3rd ed. Oxford: Oxford University Press, pp. 457–490.

Index